TEXTBOOK OF
CONTRACEPTIVE PRACTICE

TEXTBOOK OF CONTRACEPTIVE PRACTICE

by JOHN PEEL
Senior Lecturer in Sociology,
University of York

& MALCOLM POTTS
Medical Director,
International Planned Parenthood Federation,
and Sometime Fellow of Sidney Sussex College,
Cambridge

CAMBRIDGE

AT THE UNIVERSITY PRESS · 1970

Published by the Syndics of the Cambridge University Press
Bentley House, 200 Euston Road, London N.W.1
American Branch: 32 East 57th Street, New York, N.Y.10022

© Cambridge University Press 1969

Library of Congress Catalogue Card Number 69–19380

International Standard Book Numbers:
0 521 07515 7 clothbound
0 521 09598 0 paperback

First published 1969
Reprinted with corrections 1970

Printed in Great Britain
at the University Printing House, Cambridge
(Brooke Crutchley, University Printer)

To our children—planned and unplanned

CONTENTS

CONTENTS

FOREWORD

by Professor Sir Dugald Baird, M.D., F.R.C.O.G.

The publication of this comprehensive and authoritative textbook is most important at this stage of man's conquest of his environment, when it is being recognized that control of population is vital for his survival. In primitive societies high fertility was kept in check by high death rates and a short lifespan. By control of disease and advances in technology death rates have been dramatically reduced and food supplies have been increased so that a higher standard of health, education and quality of life is possible, provided population increase is not allowed to outrun supplies and services. The poorest two-thirds of the world are increasing at the fastest rate and the most urgent question today is how can the poorly educated and depressed people of these countries be motivated to carry through a programme of contraception?

The problem is not so massive in the richer countries such as Britain but it has not been entirely solved. The perfect contraceptive has not been found and there is still the problem of the social class differential in practising effective birth control. In addition there is still a failure to recognize that responsible planned parenthood is a moral duty.

This book deals with the history of contraception and it is salutary to be reminded how as recently as 30 years ago the whole idea of contraception was frowned upon in Britain, even by the medical profession, with a few notable exceptions such as Lord Dawson of Penn, whose public support of birth control did much to overcome resistance to its use. Today the situation has been transformed, although there are still those who make false distinctions between 'social' and 'medical' grounds for the approved use of contraception. In Britain today an average of less than 2·5 children per family is sufficient to secure replacement of the population and the family doctor must assume more responsibility for advising parents on contraceptive methods and indeed on many socio-sexual problems which are important to the health of the whole family.

The book gives a detailed description of available methods, including sterilization and abortion and contains much practical advice which will be welcomed by doctors and nurses. It is extremely well written, easy to read, scientifically accurate and displays a compassionate view of a human problem. No doubt this is a product of the new association of medicine and sociology which is leading to a better understanding of the world in which we live and of the way our environment affects health and behaviour.

PREFACE

This book is an attempt to bring together the most important and up to date information on clinical and sociological aspects of the control of fertility—contraception, sterilization and abortion. It is a response to the growing professional interest in all branches of the subject and it is especially intended for use in undergraduate and post-graduate courses in family planning which are forming an increasingly important part of medical education in Britain and in the United States. The Royal College of Obstetricians and Gynaecologists has recently decided to include this topic in its syllabus for the D.Obst. examination, a majority of British medical schools now provide some basic teaching on family planning and the organizers of refresher courses for general practitioners have discovered a lively demand for information on contraception. In the United States the American Medical Association adopted a report from its Committee on Human Reproduction in 1964 which emphasised the central role of the physician in family planning and the need for adequate training in contraceptive techniques and amongst the official policy statements adopted by the AMA is one that states: 'An intelligent recognition of the problems that relate to human reproduction, including the need for population control, is more than a matter of responsible parenthood: it is a matter of responsible medical practice.' For all doctors and medical students, as well as for nurses, midwives and health visitors, this book should be of value.

The subject is being introduced into the medical curriculum in the context of preventive and social medicine and it was therefore considered appropriate that this volume should be a collaborative undertaking by a clinician and a sociologist and that it should stress the cultural and epi-demiological, as well as the more strictly medical implications, of the subject. For this reason the book will be of interest to social workers and social science students for whom the problem of hyperfertility is of such central importance. And despite the fact that this book does *not* contain any exposition of the elementary facts of the physiology of reproduction, we expect that the intelligent layman will find much to interest him in virtually every chapter.

There is an urgent need to improve the standard of family planning practice in western countries—not only because it is an important part of medical care but because improvements in contraceptive technology and the acquisition of a body of skilled workers are more important than mere financial aid in strengthening the family planning services of developing countries. Thus, whether directly or indirectly, we hope that this book will contribute to the attempts which are being made to cope with the problem of world population growth. For although it is primarily about family planning in Europe and America it includes an evaluation of methods and projects which have been found to be effective in other countries. Unlike most writers, however, we have not assumed that those techniques which have attracted clinical approval, though minority usage, in western societies are necessarily those which will contribute most substantially to the growth of family limitation elsewhere. Thus, the widely used, yet inadequately studied, techniques of coitus interruptus and the condom are fully discussed and considerable attention is given to a realistic evaluation of the role of abortion, to the techniques by which it is performed and to an assessment of the mortality and morbidity rates associated with this and other forms of fertility control.

We believe the case for fertility control, by whatever means, to be socially and medically self-evident and we are, despite recent events within the Catholic church, encouraged to think that an increasing number of people are coming to share this viewpoint. Consequently, instead of discussing the so-called 'ethics' of birth control we have described the prevailing legal framework as it applies to all aspects of family limitation in different countries of the world and have attempted to assess the likely effects of the many recent and proposed changes in the law and administration. We have also tried to evaluate the role of the medical practitioner in this rapidly changing social and legal situation.

The Agreed Test for chemical spermicides which forms Appendix I first appeared in the I.P.P.F.'s *Medical Handbook* and is reprinted by permission of the Federation. Parts of chapters one and two have previously been published in *Population Studies* and we are grateful to the joint editors of that journal for allowing us to include them here. The extracts from BS 3704:1964 on the testing of rubber condoms are reproduced in Appendix II by permission of the British Standards

Institution, 2 Park Street, London w.1, from whom copies of the complete standard may be obtained.

We are indebted to Peter Cox, Rodney Dale, Peter Diggory, Alan Guttmacher and Miss Dorothea Kerslake for helpful comments on the whole, or on specific chapters, of the manuscript and to others who have provided valuable comment or assisted in various ways in the preparation of this book. We owe a special debt to Sir Dugald Baird for his encouragement, criticisms and suggestions and for his kindness in writing a Foreword. The responsibility for the final text, and for any shortcomings, is of course our own.

JOHN PEEL

MALCOLM POTTS

Cambridge
November 1968

1 THE MEDICAL HISTORY OF CONTRACEPTION

BIRTH CONTROL'S PRE-HISTORY

Birth control practice is today regarded by a substantial and influential majority of doctors as an important element in preventive medicine and the provision of contraceptive advice an appropriate activity for the medical practitioner. This viewpoint is, however, a product of the last 40 years and its adoption represents one of the major achievements of the English birth control movement and its international extensions whose early activities were directed as much towards the indifference of the medical profession as against the hostility of religious groups and public opinion.

In societies of antiquity contraceptive knowledge had a written basis in texts which formed a continuous medical tradition from the works of Aristotle in the fourth century B.C., through a variety of Greek and Roman authors, to Pliny the Elder and Dioscorides in the first century A.D. In the second century Soranus, a Greek doctor practising in Rome, advanced in his *Gynaecia* both technique and theory to a level surpassed only during the last 60 years, and after him the tradition was continued in the work of Caelius Aurelianus in the fifth century and of Aetius in the sixth. Certainly such clinical knowledge was never widely diffused and in most of these writings rational techniques were discussed alongside magical recipes. Nevertheless, it was from this continuous tradition that the contraceptive methods which were to be popularized in Europe during the nineteenth and twentieth centuries were derived, though the derivation was secondary and via Islamic sources.

Medical theory and practice in mediaeval Europe were developed within the ethos of the Catholic Church and medical education was undertaken largely as an adjunct of monastic learning.[1] In these circumstances the neglect of contraceptive practice by pre-nineteenth-century physicians is hardly surprising. Indeed, when Soranus's *Gynaecia* was eventually resurrected and transcribed the contraceptive passages were

I

entirely omitted[2] and even amongst English writers on syphilology there was a reluctance to discuss the condom, well known since the sixteenth century as a prophylactic against venereal infection. John Marten (1702) referred to Saxonia's impregnated linen sheath but refused to divulge the composition of the wash 'lest it give encouragement to the lewd' and Joseph Cam (1734) declared that 'to publish methods of prevention smells so rank of the libertine and freethinker that it ought not to be allowed in a Christian country'.

THE EARLY NINETEENTH-CENTURY BIRTH CONTROL MOVEMENT

The pioneers of the nineteenth-century birth control movement, which arose in response to the debate on Malthus's famous *Essay on Population*, nevertheless assumed a medical responsibility in the provision of contraceptive advice. Although the appeal of Francis Place's 'Diabolical Handbills' (perhaps the earliest vehicle of domiciliary birth control advice, in the distribution of which the young John Stuart Mill became entangled with the police) was primarily economic, in one edition constitutional weaknesses and pelvic malformation were specified as therapeutic indications for birth control: a point of view which did not find its way into the medical press for another 100 years. Place records that, in framing his handbills, he sought the advice of physicians and claims that the methods recommended had the approval of 'accouchers of the first respectability and surgeons of great eminence', and though he provides no clue to their identity it is known that Place was a close friend of Thomas Wakley, the medical reformer who founded and for many years edited the *Lancet*.

Yet, despite an increasing concern in nineteenth-century Britain with the problems of infant and maternal mortality and morbidity, of induced abortion and infanticide, medical opinion succeeded in ignoring the birth control issue for the next 40 years. The only English contribution to the literature in this period[3] went unnoticed in the medical press and its author's discretion in publishing pseudonymously was to be fully justified by subsequent events. The discussion of technique in this particular work (though Drysdale was a venereologist of some repute) was not more noticeably rigorous than in contemporary non-medical publications and it is doubtful whether the physiology of reproduction was yet sufficiently understood to have facilitated any significant advance in contraceptive theory. In the meantime the medical press maintained an attitude of indifference which is illustrated by a correspondent writing in the *Lancet* in 1859: 'It often occurs to me in reading cases where women whose pelvices have become distorted by mollitis ossium, are delivered of dead or mutilated children, that the question involves a consideration apart from a medical one. If a woman is aware that her pelvis is so deformed that it is physically impossible that anything can pass through it and retain life, why is she at liberty to continue connexion with her husband when she knows the inevitable consequences will be the destruction of her child? Would it not be a merciful act to place a penalty upon that woman's becoming pregnant again, being morally on her part a case of murder? A woman knowing this, and persisting in sexual congress is really as guilty as the woman who destroys her child after it is born.' Seven years later the Harveian Society's Committee on Infanticide was unable to proceed beyond the assumption that the victims of the practice were 'mostly the illegitimate offspring of domestic servants' and, in spite of Drysdale's influence as secretary of the Committee, its nineteen recommendations contained no hint of birth control as a preventive measure.

When in the late 1860s it became apparent that the subject could no longer be ignored the medical profession's indifference gave way to vigorous opposition. The official organs of the profession were provoked into their first explicit mention of contraception by the Amberley incident in 1868.[4] Lord Amberley, father of Bertrand Russell, presided over a meeting of the London Dialectical Society at which his former tutor, James Laurie, spoke on the problem of large families and at which Charles Bradlaugh and Drysdale also spoke. In summing up, Amberley deplored the attitude of the church to the subject of birth control but expressed the hope that medical men would have something to contribute through the discussion of innocuous methods. The *British Medical Journal* reported with satisfaction that one of the medical men who had attended the meeting 'wishes us to intimate that he would not by any means be a party to assigning to the profession any such anti-genetic function' and the *Medical Times and Gazette* deplored Lord Amberley's 'most scandalous insult' to the medical profession. At the annual meeting of the BMA the following year Dr Beatty condemned 'the beastly contrivances for limiting the numbers of offspring' and in commending these comments the *Lancet* commented: 'We do not think that the practices to which we have been compelled to refer would be tolerated even as subjects for discussion by more than a very small number of medical men; but these have contrived to obtain a wide publicity for their peculiar views.'

THE MALTHUSIAN LEAGUE

The Malthusian League, established after the famous Bradlaugh–Besant trial of 1877 (see chapter 2), was the forerunner of the modern birth control movement, and recognized the need to transform English medical opinion on this subject. In 1880 a Medical and Scientific Branch of the League was formed on the initiative of Drysdale and a Leeds physician, H. A. Allbutt, in order to obtain for the League the support of the medical profession 'the weight of whose influence will be such as to gain for the principles of neo-Malthusians the respect and, ultimately, the adherence of all thoughtful people'. Although it was responsible for organizing, in 1881, the first international medical conference on birth control which was attended by more than forty practitioners from various European countries, the medical branch never attracted more than a handful of English doctors and its influence on professional opinion can only have been damaged by the Allbutt incident of 1887.

Allbutt, who was by this time secretary of the League's medical branch, appeared before the General Medical Council on the charge of having 'published and exposed for sale an indecent publication entitled *The Wife's Handbook*, and having published and attached thereto advertisements of an unprofessional character titled "Malthusian Appliances"'. The Council found against Allbutt and erased his name from the Register. In fact, *The Wife's Handbook* was an inoffensive little manual on domestic hygiene which included chapters on ante-natal care, pregnancy and the management of the baby, in addition to the chapter on 'How to Prevent Conception'. A clinically significant feature of the discussion under this last heading was the mention, for the first time in an English publication, of the Mensinga diaphragm about which Allbutt had presumably learned from the Dutch delegates to the international conference. The use of the impregnated sponge, the condom, douching and the use of Rendell's quinine pessaries were fully described. Coitus interruptus was described as a 'method advocated by many eminent physicians' but the safe period, for which a 95 per cent success rate was claimed, was erroneously described as lying between the ninth and twenty-third days of the cycle!

The General Medical Council's treatment of Allbutt undoubtedly delayed the development of a favourable medical attitude to birth control in England. In contrast, American medical journals had, from the 1880s, carried articles in which both the desirability of family limitation and the relative merits of different contraceptive techniques were rationally discussed. In the United States an active birth control movement had been initiated in the 1830s by Robert Dale Owen, son of the English co-operative pioneer, and Dr Charles Knowlton. Robert Owen's *Moral Physiology* (1830) was the first book on birth control to be published in America and Knowlton's *Fruits of Philosophy* (1832) was perhaps the most influential contraceptive pamphlet ever to appear. Technically, it was an advance on anything which had appeared before and superior to almost anything which appeared during the next 50 years; it circulated widely in the United States and, most important of all, it was this pamphlet which, in its English edition, was the subject of the notorious Bradlaugh–Besant trial in 1877.

In America, as in England, the birth control movement attracted a number of eccentric protagonists but, unlike its English counterpart, it had the firm support of a number of eminent doctors including A. M. Mauriceau, R. T. Trall, Edward Bliss Foote, Edward Bond Foote and Alice B. Stockham. The Comstock Act of 1873, which prohibited the distribution through the mails of contraceptive information, and the prosecutions which took place under its provisions induced a certain caution amongst most members of the medical profession but did not prevent the journals from publishing articles on contraception. The earliest of these was the 1882 issue of the *Michigan Medical News* and in 1888 the *Medical and Surgical Reporter* produced a symposium number devoted to contraception. Although they contributed little to the advancement of technique the articles in this issue were notable for their enlightened attitude to a practice which was acknowledged to be widely employed.

The English medical press continued to condemn the practice editorially and to publicize every expression of the anti-birth control point of view for another 40 years. The grounds for opposition to contraception were basically ethical and moral, the use of such adjectives as 'lustful', 'selfish' and 'immoral' being obligatory in any mention of the subject. In addition, however, doctors now began to stress the alleged harmful physical effects of contraception, effects which included galloping cancer, sterility and nymphomania in women and mental decay, amnesia and cardiac palpitations in men; in both sexes the practice was likely to produce mania leading to suicide.[5] Moral and clinical objections occasionally converged as, for example, in the *Lancet* editorial which described contraception as 'a sin against physiology', and there was a noticeable tendency to confuse abortion and contraception.

It has been suggested[6] that, despite this ostensible attitude to contraception, the idea of family limitation was gaining increasing acceptance amongst individual practitioners. Certainly doctors had been one of the earliest social groups to restrict their own fertility (see chapter 2) and in evidence before the National Birth Rate Commission in 1914 it was stated that it had by then become 'almost a rule' for doctors to advocate the spacing of pregnancies. It was not claimed that doctors were in the habit of advising on the means to be adopted and the evidence is that either abstinence was enjoined or that parents were left to discover a method for themselves amongst the variety of commercial products then available. To these the attitude of the majority of doctors remained uncompromising; in 1905 the south-western branch of the British Medical Association passed a resolution condemning the growing use of 'ecbolics and contraceptives' and four years later the parent Association supported Lord Braye's bill which aimed at outlawing the sale of contraceptives.

Despairing at this lack of medical leadership, the Malthusian League, which since the Allbutt incident had confined its activities to publicizing the economic and social advantages of family limitation, decided in 1913 to enter the field of medical propaganda. This it was encouraged to do by the fact that Sir James Barr, in his presidential address to the BMA in the previous year, had not only advocated a low birth rate on eugenic grounds but had also omitted the expected ritual condemnation of contraception! In launching its practical leaflet the League declared: 'The Council of the Malthusian League, while continuing to regard this as a matter which is strictly within the province of the medical profession and which ought to be taken over by them, has compiled a leaflet entitled *Hygienic Methods of Family Limitation*, for the benefit of those desirous of limiting their families but who are ignorant of the means of doing so and unable to get medical advice on the subject.' In spite of the careful restrictions placed on its distribution this pamphlet had a wide circulation and underwent numerous revisions. More than 3,000 copies were applied for during the first year of publication and 200 doctors were included amongst the applicants. This was the only medical birth control publication to appear during the first 20 years of the present century and though it contained a useful review of existing techniques it contributed little to contraceptive theory. It was by now apparent to the League that this could only be advanced by the establishment of birth control clinics 'along the lines of those operating in Holland' and this proposal was widely canvassed in neo-Malthusian discussion from 1913 onwards. The First World War intervened, however, and the 'first birth control clinic in the British Empire', as its founder characteristically described it, was established by Marie Stopes in 1921, a few months before the opening of the first of the League's clinics, at Walworth.

EARLY TWENTIETH-CENTURY TRANSITION

By this time general attitudes to the birth control question had become so vocal that the medical profession could not for long ignore the issue. The influence of war as a solvent of public prejudice has frequently been remarked upon; the transformation of attitudes to sexual questions generally and to birth control specifically during the period of the First World War is an event without parallel in English social history. The concessions to feminism, a growing concern with infant and maternal mortality, the first open discussion of venereal disease, the literary impact of Freud, Lawrence, Carpenter and Joyce; above all, the influence of Havelock Ellis whose *Studies in the Psychology of Sex*, banned as a 'bawdy, scandalous and obscene libel' in the nineties, became the 'classic and dictionary of the twenties'—these were amongst the factors which contributed to the enlightenment of public discussion within which the personal and social importance of family limitation was now clearly recognized. Slowly and reluctantly, the doctors responded to this changed outlook. By carefully distinguishing between contraception and abortion and by pointing to the complete absence of evidence for the supposed injurious effects of contraceptive usage, the 1916 Report of the National Birth Rate Commission had provided reassurance, at least for the more responsible sections of the profession, on the two most frequent objections to the practice. Both objections continued to appear but it was now conceded that some contraceptives were probably less harmful than others. Moreover, the equation of contraception and abortion was more often insinuated, e.g. by suggesting that two practitioners should be required to give approval to the use of contraceptives, than taken for granted. When this suggestion was advanced by a gynaecologist at a meeting of the Medico-Legal Society, Earl Russell pointed out that 'it would be embarrassing and expensive to have to use contraceptives only in the presence of two members of the medical profession'. The journals, however, were now prepared to drop their opposition to birth control; after a 'last ditch' attempt to argue that contraceptives were notoriously unable to prevent conception,[7] the subject virtually disappeared from the pages of the *Lancet* and the *British Medical Journal*. Both published favourable reviews of Marie Stopes' *Married Love* in 1919 but omitted reference to the passages on birth control; her subsequent volume, *Wise Parenthood*, which developed the subject more fully was advertised on the front page of the *Lancet*.

Meanwhile, a number of prominent doctors were beginning openly to advocate family limitation and there is evidence that within the profession as a whole there was less hostility than had been supposed. In a lecture on 'The Problem of Birth Control', given before the Royal Institute of Public Health in 1918, Dr Killick Millard, Medical Officer of Health for Leicester, stressed the desirability of birth control on public health grounds and revealed that he had recently asked 80 doctors for their views on this question. Six had pleaded lack of knowledge and of the rest 'those who regarded birth control as being harmless were five times the more numerous'. Three years later Millard conducted a second enquiry, this time amongst gynaecologists and women doctors, to whom 160 questionnaires were sent, 65 being returned. To the substantive questions the following replies were obtained:

Question 1 'Do you approve of married couples using contraceptive methods in cases where, on health or economic grounds, they feel it incumbent on them to limit the size of the family?'

37 answered 'Yes'   13 answered 'No'

14 gave a qualified approval, e.g. only after one, two or three children; only on medical advice; on health grounds only (6 replies).

Question 2 'If so, which method or methods do you consider, on the whole, to be most satisfactory?'

Answers

18 Condom	2 Douching
5 Condom or some other method	2 'Observing the periods'
8 Quinine pessaries	1 Vaginal plug
3 Check pessary	1 Various
1 Check pessary plus quinine pessary	17 Not stated
2 Coitus interruptus	3 Abstinence
	2 Abstinence or condom

Although, as Millard suggested in presenting these results, it could no longer be claimed that doctors condemned contraception, the low response rate was an indication of a widespread reluctance even to have the subject discussed; moreover, some of the incidental observations which Millard had invited on his questionnaire revealed a continuing concern with its possible physical and moral consequences. The answers to the question on methods are almost certainly more indicative of the respondents' own domestic preferences than of any attempted evaluation. The lack of support for the check pessary, in view of the profession's subsequent partiality for the device, is remarkable.

One of the most important events in the twentieth-century history of birth control was the outspoken address by Lord Dawson of Penn to the 1921 Church Congress at Birmingham. Dawson was by no means a recent convert to family limitation; whilst still a medical student he had courageously signed a petition to the General Medical Council protesting at its treatment of Allbutt in 1887[8] and, with a number of other students had written and distributed a practical birth control tract, *Few in the Family*, *Happiness at Home*. His Birmingham speech was a reasoned defence of 'artificial birth control' on medical, social and, especially, personal grounds; he challenged the more common objections to the practice, condemned abstention as 'pernicious' and called on the Church to revise its opinions on sexual matters in the light of modern knowledge. It would be difficult to exaggerate the effect of this speech on public opinion. 'Probably no utterance of recent times', declared the *Malthusian*, 'has so profoundly stirred the press and public as this outspoken declaration from such a high authority, and it has called forth a plethora of comment, mostly favourable, from the daily press, medical and clerical authorities and eugenists.' As the King's physician, Dawson had virtually put the monarchy on the side of family limitation; his choice of platform, moreover, in view of the predominantly moral and religious objections to birth control, was an appropriate one and the press responded accordingly. The *Sunday Express* (headline: 'Lord Dawson Must Go') was almost alone amongst national newspapers in condemning the speech and the response of the medical journals was hardly less enthusiastic. 'The interest aroused by Lord Dawson's courageous address', wrote the editor of the *Lancet*, 'makes the gap in medical knowledge a very noticeable one, and steps are already being taken at least to take stock of the present position. The Federation of Medical

9

Women chose this subject for consideration at their first meeting this session. . . The Federation of Medical and Allied Societies are discussing the question. . . and we commend the subject to the consideration of other medical societies.' 'A joint meeting of gynaecologists and neurologists', it was whimsically suggested, 'might clear the ground of some of its rough places.' The contemporary issue of the *British Medical Journal* broke entirely new ground by summarizing, for the first time in a medical paper, the practical methods of contraception discussed at the Medical Women's conference.

During the next few years a great deal was written by doctors on the subject of contraception, much of it of an indifferent quality. Even by the standards of 40 years ago, the majority of the articles published in the special contraception issue of 'The Leading Medical Monthly Journal' in 1923 reveals an almost incredible lack of objectivity. Amongst the ten authors contributing to this issue, only Norman Haire, who had experience as medical consultant to the Malthusian League's Walworth clinic, managed to rise above the level of mediocrity. Of the rest, all distinguished consulting gynaecologists or obstetricians, three asserted that contraceptive usage produced sterility, a fourth alleged mental degeneration in subsequent offspring and a fifth equated birth control with masturbation as a practice 'distinctly dangerous to health'. All of them backed up their obviously limited medical knowledge with aphoristic moralizing, eugenic and demographic prognostications and totally unsupported generalizations regarding parental motivation. A symposium by nine different but equally eminent doctors published three years later[9] managed to achieve an even more uniform level of banality. This was introduced by Sir Thomas Horder as 'the sort of scientific enquiry that the subject needs'; in fact most of the writers were opponents of birth control and not one was prepared to adopt even the very moderate position advocated by Dawson. These two volumes were fairly typical of much of the general medical discussion of contraception during the 1920s.

It may be that, in the medical world as elsewhere, the most vocal points of view tend to be those of the extremists and that many practising doctors were behaving in a far more reasonable manner than either the radical or the conservative standpoints openly expressed would suggest. Yet, in his celebrated medical novel of this period,[10] Cronin provides what is presumably intended to represent the attitude of the family doctor. Though Manson, the doctor-hero, is portrayed as an enlightened and progressive young physician, struggling against the bigotry and humbug of his profession, he is nevertheless revolted when asked by the local minister for contraceptive advice.

THE BIRTH CONTROL INVESTIGATION COMMITTEE

The Report of the Medical Committee of the National Birth Rate Commission of 1927 drew attention to the lack of scientific knowledge of the efficiency of contraceptives and to the need for systematic collection of statistical data over a period of years.

It was with the object of providing this sort of scientific data, on which more adequate medical guidance could be based, that the Birth Control Investigation Committee was established in 1927. This organization developed out of the predominantly lay-inspired voluntary clinic movement which, by this date, was operating 12 clinics in England and Scotland. Of these, the most important were the nine affiliated to the Society for the Provision of Birth Control Clinics (SPBCC) which, by the end of 1927, had collectively dealt with 13,000 new patients and 17,000 return cases. At each of these clinics the recommended method of contraception was the spring-rim vaginal diaphragm, fitted initially by a doctor, and subsequently used in combination with a spermicidal jelly and douching. This procedure, adopted in the early, heroic days, when a concern for maximum safety was an overriding consideration, was increasingly felt to be too elaborate for many of the clinics' clientele and follow-up visits to non-returning patients revealed that large numbers of these had not been able to persevere with the method.[11] The complete lack of factual information prompted the formation of a group under the Chairmanship of Sir Humphry Rolleston, which christened itself the Birth Control Investigation Committee (BCIC). Its joint secretaries were the Hon. Mrs Marjorie Farrer and Dr C. P. Blacker, later general secretary of the Eugenics Society. Its objects were 'to investigate the sociological and medical principles of contraception; the possible effects of the practice on physical and mental health; and the merits and demerits of all possible methods'. During the 12 years of its existence this Committee, with generous financial support from the Eugenics Society, carried out an ambitious and comprehensive research programme on social and clinical aspects of contraception. Blacker was Secretary both of the BCIC and of the International Medical Group for the Investigation of Birth Control and the reports of the former were given an added dimension through their incorporation in the yearly publications of the International Group.

The early statistical work of the BCIC was concerned with the analysis of information obtained at the birth control clinics; this provided useful data on the social composition and previous contraceptive histories of the clinic clientele and on the effectiveness and acceptability of the contraceptive methods in use. The long-term results of this work were seen in a more self-critical attitude on the part of the clinic personnel who showed a greater attention to methods of recording and a concern with the problem of the non-persistent patient. It was realized, however, that the investigations conducted on clinic patients were limited to selected social groups and the Committee therefore undertook a survey designed to obtain information on the contraceptive practices of the general public. This was based on 500 completed postal questionnaires, and despite its acknowledged limitations, it was superior to any work previously undertaken. Harold Laski, in his foreword to the volume in which the results of this survey were published,[12] was able to comment: 'Books like this are a happy proof that the birth control movement is passing rapidly from the stage of enthusiasm to the stage of science.'

In the clinical field, the BCIC sponsored or financially supported a large number of research projects on contraception and allied problems. These included:

(i) Investigations at Oxford by Dr H. M. Carlton and Professor Howard Florey on uterine action during coitus.[13]

(ii) A literature survey on the artificial production of sterility by the use of spermatoxins by Dr C. F. Cosin.[14]

(iii) Investigations by Dr H. M. Carlton and Dr H. J. Phelps into the effectiveness of intra-uterine pessaries.[15]

(iv) Early experimental work by Dr B. P. Wiesner at Edinburgh on hormonal interference with ovulation and pregnancy.[16]

(v) Investigations at Oxford by Dr Solly Zuckerman on periodicity in the fertility of primates and the deposition of estrogens on the sexual skin of monkeys.[17]

The most exhaustive and significant project, however, was the research carried out at Oxford by Dr J. R. Baker and his colleagues into chemical contraception. Besides contributing to the fundamental theory of contraception,[18] this work led to the elaboration of Volpar, one of the most important advances in the pre-hormonal history of contraception, to the elaboration of tests of spermicidal activity and to the first independent assessment of commercial contraceptives.

Much of the work of the BCIC had to be carried out on the periphery of established medical research. Wiesner's work at the University of Edinburgh was done in the Animal Breeding Research Department where Professor F. A. E. Crew had already provided facilities for work sponsored by the US birth control movement. At the University of Oxford Baker had begun his research in the Department of Zoology but when the nature of his investigations was discovered by the Professor of Zoology he was denied the further use of laboratories in that Department; the whole project would have ended or been seriously impeded if Professor Howard Florey (later Lord Florey, President of the Royal Society) had not immediately offered Baker laboratory facilities in the Department of Pathology. For Baker, contraceptive research in the 1920s is permanently symbolized in his recollection of assembling his apparatus and reagents on a handcart and trundling this from department to department, through the streets of Oxford.[19] In such an atmosphere, the BCIC made a unique contribution to the improved status of contraception in medical circles both by its influence on clinic procedure and through the undoubted quality of its original research, the results of which were accepted without demur by the professional journals. In 1930, when the SPBCC was reconstituted as the National Birth Control Association, medical opinion had been sufficiently transformed to allow Sir Thomas Horder to become its first President.

THE BIRTH CONTROL CLINIC MOVEMENT

In the same year, contraception attained a legitimate and permanent place in preventive medicine through the publication of the Ministry of Health's Memorandum 153 MCW which empowered local authorities to provide birth control advice to limited classes of women when this was necessitated by exclusively medical circumstances. This memorandum, the outcome of years of lay pressure on successive ministers and the only governmental concession to the birth control movement in this country until the 1967 Family Planning Act, once again exposed the deficiencies of the medical profession. Within a year 36 authorities had taken action under its provisions but, due to the general lack of contraceptive expertise amongst their own medical staffs, the majority were obliged to refer their patients to the voluntary clinics. The latter, from the outset, performed an important secondary function in training doctors in contraceptive techniques, though in this they were handicapped by their failure to obtain adequate publicity in the medical press. The *British Medical Journal*, for example, was still refusing advertisements for Marie Stopes' doctors' session in 1932.

Nor is it surprising, given the prevailing medical attitudes, that the early voluntary clinics had difficulty in obtaining the services of doctors and in retaining these once the local BMA branch had learned of their activities. It was particularly hazardous for the woman doctor, whose position within the profession was still a precarious one, to risk association with such a dubious enterprise. Moreover, the medical role in clinic organization was characterized by a number of quite unusual features which were a potential source of resentment by the profession.

Clinic doctors were employed by lay committees from whose policy deliberations they were frequently excluded (the FPA's model branch constitution provides for the attendance of clinic doctors at Committee meetings in an advisory capacity and recommends that their advice be sought when clinic procedure is being discussed); yet the responsibility for clinic practice rested solely with the doctor. Quite apart from the dangers of litigation in a period when any number of doctors could be persuaded to attribute almost any ailment to the use of contraceptives, there were many other matters on which lay and professional attitudes were likely to conflict. (In 1926 the Committee of the North Kensington Clinic decided that in cases where the contraceptive appliance supplied to a patient had failed the cost should be refunded. This was rescinded however when the clinic doctors objected that 'usually, in the case of failure the fault can be traced to some omission on the part of the patient'.) Nor were such differences easily resolved in the emotionally charged atmosphere of the early clinics. For if the lay workers had a devotion to their 'cause' and to their clinics, the doctors too had emotional motivations for the work they were doing and a personal commitment to their patients.

An additional handicap for the clinic doctor arose out of the contravention of medical etiquette which her work in the clinic represented. An accepted rule of the medical profession, to which few exceptions are made, is that a doctor will not treat another doctor's patient, except at the latter's request or in an emergency, and that if he does (by request, in emergency or inadvertently) he informs his colleague as early as possible. The work of the clinics clearly involved a complete breach of this convention; indeed, since they were founded on the assumption that the majority of private practitioners were opposed to the use of contraceptives, it would have been clearly impossible for the clinics to have fulfilled the requirements of professional etiquette in this way. In 1926 the Aberdeen clinic was disaffiliated from the Society for the Provision of Birth Control Clinics for insisting on exercising precisely this convention and was re-admitted to membership only after it had rescinded the relevant rule.[20] This particular difficulty has never been clarified although it was the subject of discussion between the Family Planning Association and the BMA as recently as 1947. The statement, in the FPA's *Speakers' Notes*[21] that 'Wherever possible the general practitioner is informed of clinic recommendations' is clearly an overstatement of the true position. This is revealed elsewhere, perhaps with unconscious irony, in the admission that 'professional relations between clinic doctors and the general practitioners is very good in many areas and is improving in most'.

DEVELOPMENTS IN THE UNITED STATES

Marie Stopes was thwarted in her undoubted ambition to found the 'first birth control clinic in the world' by developments in the United States which, in the early decades of the present century, provide a strange parallel with events in England. In 1921, the same year in which Sir James Barr cautiously commended the benefits of birth restriction to his British medical colleagues, Dr Abraham Jacobi, in his presidential address to the American Medical Association, unequivocally advocated the use of contraception on economic, social and medical grounds. But just as the task of public advocacy of family limitation in England fell largely to lay enthusiasts like Marie Stopes and the pioneers of the SPBCC, in America too the central figure in organizing an active birth control movement was Mrs Margaret Sanger.

Margaret Sanger's 'fight for birth control' (the title of her autobiography)[22] took many forms including a plan to flood the country with a million copies of her pamphlet *Family Limitation*, a subsequent flight to Europe where she visited Holland and learned of the Mensinga diaphragm and—most important of all—the establishment of the first birth control advice centre at Brooklyn in 1916. Although this was quickly closed down as a public nuisance by the New York police it represented a genuine milestone in contraceptive history.

Fortunately, Mrs Sanger had an extraordinary capacity for dramatic presentation of her theme. She persisted with the Brooklyn clinic and, though she served a term of imprisonment, eventually secured a decision[23] in the Court of Appeals which enabled medically qualified personnel to give contraceptive advice legally 'for the cure and prevention of disease', a phrase which was liberally interpreted. Margaret Sanger was also one of the architects of the international family planning movement. In 1927 she organized, in Geneva, the first World Population Conference which was attended by leading scientists, sociologists and doctors from Europe and America. This resulted in the formation of two important committees, the International Medical Group (see p. 11) and the International Union for the Scientific Study of Population, which has survived as the official association of professional demographers. In 1948 Mrs Sanger brought together delegates from 23 countries to form the organization which subsequently became the International Planned Parenthood Federation of which she was formerly President Emeritus.

In her attitude to the medical profession Mrs. Sanger was closer to the Society for the Provision of Birth Control Clinics than to Marie Stopes, who ignored and often alienated doctors. Mrs Sanger deliberately set out to co-operate with the more enlightened sections of the profession and amongst her early and most distinguished associates were Dr R. L. Dickinson and Drs Abraham and Hannah Stone. As president of the American Gynecological Society in 1920 Dickinson pleaded for more research on contraceptive techniques and three years later published the first authoritative medical article on contraception which he posted to physicians all over the country in order to challenge the Comstock Act. Dickinson founded, and was for a number of years secretary to the National Committee on Maternal Health, an organization carrying out (though on a more extensive scale) broadly similar activities to Blacker's Birth Control Investigation Committee and financing much fundamental research in the US and in England.

Abraham Stone edited the first medical journal devoted to contraception: the *Journal of Contraception* which first appeared in 1935. In addition, with the sociologist Norman Himes, he was co-author of what was for many years the standard birth control textbook.[24] His wife made a singular contribution to the development of family planning by importing, in 1936, a package of contraceptive materials (see p. 213) and in the course of the protracted legal proceedings which followed succeeded in removing the 'federal handcuffs shackling the medical prescription of contraception'.[25]

In spite of the greater formal restrictions imposed by legislation, family planning in the United States has not had less distinguished medical support than in Britain. The growth of birth control clinics has been slower and more modest; the voluntary clinics see about the same number of patients each year as in Britain. But the Planned Parenthood Federation of America and associated organizations have made fundamental contributions to the development of contraceptive practice which have had a truly international significance. Moreover, in 1959 family planning received official medical endorsement in a resolution of the American Public Health Association which was subsequently confirmed by the American College of Obstetricians and Gynecologists.

THE FUTURE

During the last ten years a number of factors have brought about significant changes in general medical attitudes to contraception in both America and Britain. In the first place the advent of the oral contraceptive—with its first generation, second generation, sequential and serial forms—has provided the doctor with a therapeutic agent which clearly justifies his professional concern. Secondly, within the profession as a whole there is now a greater emphasis on preventive medicine whilst the general practitioner is increasingly accepting responsibility for a wide range of para-medical services within which the provision of contraceptive advice may be regarded as an appropriate and valuable activity. Finally the 1967 Family Planning Act, which attempts to involve local authorities very much more directly in contraceptive provision, has legitimized a situation which many doctors previously regarded as equivocal.

This changing situation has created a lag in medical education the dimensions of which are revealed in a recent survey in England. In an enquiry[26] amongst general practitioners on the Sheffield Executive Council List in April 1967 93 per cent of those doctors interviewed advised their patients directly on contraceptive matters, although only 32 per cent had received either undergraduate or postgraduate instruction in contraceptive technique. Amongst those qualified before 1950 this proportion was as low as 18 per cent rising to 56 per cent amongst those qualified after that date.

2 PATTERNS OF FAMILY PLANNING

FECUNDITY AND FERTILITY

There is no evidence that human fecundity, the biological capacity for procreation, has varied significantly either from society to society or from one century to another. Although there are wide individual differences in the biological capacity to reproduce, these appear to be fairly constantly distributed amongst human populations and the overall pattern of achieved fertility—the actual number of children produced—is more fundamentally influenced by environmental, social and psychological factors than by any basic physiological variation. As the biological extremes of sterility and hyper-fecundity are progressively mitigated, the one by subfertility treatment and the other by effective birth control practice, sociological factors become even more important determinants of achieved fertility.

Given a set of social circumstances which were uniformly favourable to maximum fertility, the average number of births per married or cohabiting woman would be about 20.[1] There is no known society in which such an average has been even remotely approached; at the 1961 Census there were only 16 women in the whole of England and Wales who had this number of children. The highest recorded average for a whole community is ten (amongst women living in rural Quebec at the time of the 1941 Census) but in most societies the average is well below six. Of course, six surviving children may be the outcome of a substantially larger number of pregnancies or births and during the major period of human existence high birth rates (though never approaching the biological limit) have been offset by high death rates.

This was the situation which prevailed in Europe during the seventeenth and eighteenth centuries and which provided Malthus with the evidence for his thesis[2] that population and food supplies were kept in equilibrium only by the natural checks of war, pestilence and famine. By the late nineteenth century, owing to better diet, improved hygiene and sanitation and advances in medical care, the death rate had fallen dramatically. An important component of this decline in mortality, illustrated in figure 1, was a reduction in neonatal and child deaths. This new imbalance in the Malthusian equation was reflected in a closing of the gap between numbers of pregnancies and size of completed family, a process which produced a new and unique type of kinship structure. The Victorian era was the first and last period in human history in which the large surviving family was the rule. Nor did it persist for more than a generation; by the late 1870s the birth rate had also started to decline and during the next 60 years mortality and fertility fell together to produce a new equilibrium (of low birth rates and low death rates) which is characteristic of all advanced societies.

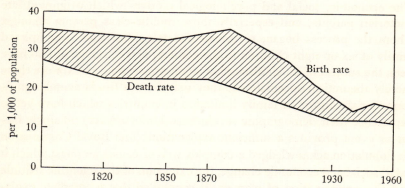

Fig. 1.   Birth and death rates, England and Wales 1790–1960.

For these trends were paralleled not only in the rest of western Europe but also in the United States where the decline began earlier and from an even larger average family size. Between 1830 and 1930 the crude birth rate, for American whites, dropped from 50 to less than 18 per thousand and, as in Britain, the fertility of those women who reached the end of their reproductive years in the 1950s was barely sufficient to maintain a stationary population.

The implications of this demographic revolution for the family structure of western societies is clearly revealed by a comparison of the proportions of different sized families which resulted from English marriages of 1860 and 1925. These figures, reproduced in table 1 from the Report of the Royal Commission on Population, relate to all women who married below the age of 45 in the specified years and who had not been widowed or divorced before the age of 45. In this relatively short

period of 65 years the proportion of families with four or more children
fell from 72 to 20 per cent and the size of completed families dropped
from an average of six to just over two.

TABLE I. *Changes in distribution of families by size*

Number of children in family	0	1	2	3	4	5	6	7	8	Over 8
Marriages of 1860 (per cent)	9	5	6	8	9	10	10	10	9	24
Marriages of 1925 (per cent)	17	25	25	14	8	5	3	2	1	1

THE RETREAT FROM PARENTHOOD

The economic, social and psychological motives which prompted late
Victorian parents, and especially those middle-class parents amongst
whom the process began, to initiate the transition from a completed
family of six or eight children to the contemporary average of two have
been the subject of much discussion amongst sociologists. Nor are these
merely theoretical speculations: they may have a fundamental significance for the future of family limitation in countries which have yet to
experience their demographic revolutions. Unfortunately no single factor or event provides a sufficient explanation. The Royal Commission
on Population acknowledged a complex web of causes amongst which it
listed social and economic change, the extension of the scientific attitude
and the emancipation of women. It concluded that a complete explanation could be discovered only by 'an unusually subtle and exhaustive
analysis of human motives and of social, economic and cultural forces'.[3]

An outstanding contribution to this analysis is to be found in Banks'
Prosperity and Parenthood[4] in which it is argued that the rising middle-
class standard of living during the late nineteenth century provided the
necessary impetus to family limitation. An increase in material prosperity, coupled with an expansion in the range of satisfactions regarded
as essential for civilized existence, had become a reality for the mid-
Victorian middle classes. But when this revolution of rising expectations
was threatened by increases in the costs of education, of domestic
servants, and of the 'paraphernalia of gentility', a retrenchment occurred. If an adequate upbringing, an expensive education and a suitable start in life were to cost more, then these privileges, instead of
being distributed more thinly amongst a large number of children,
would in future necessitate a reduction in the numbers of beneficiaries.

There were undoubtedly other threats to the established way of life which contributed to the desire of Victorian parents to limit their families. The increasing power of the trades unions, the growth of feminism and, above all, the challenge to religious values and beliefs which the expansion and popularization of scientific, especially biological, ideas entailed: all these represented an undermining of the assumptions on which middle-class prosperity was based. Nor can the physiological burdens of pregnancy and childbearing have been entirely irrelevant to the decision to restrict family size. The fatalism with which Queen Victoria regarded[5] the discomforts of motherhood ('God's will be done and if He decrees that we are to have a great number of children, why we must try to bring them up as useful and exemplary members of society') had now given way to a demand for emancipation from domestic, as well as political, legal and social, restrictions.

The process of family limitation in western societies began amongst the upper-middle and middle classes; doctors and clergymen were, according to the 1911 Census,[6] the earliest occupational groups to limit their families, closely followed by teachers. But as the economic advantages of the small family became apparent, broader sections of the population began to adopt the practices of those in the class immediately above them. This process of social emulation was relatively slow and was never carried to completion but the Victorian middle-class family's choice between a third child or a carriage and pair had its equivalent in the alternatives, confronting the suburban family of the 1930s, of a baby or a baby Austin. In this way the two-child family norm became firmly established though the success with which individual families were able to conform to this ideal continued to vary inversely with social class.

THE BRADLAUGH–BESANT TRIAL

If the underlying causes of the desire for family limitation are obscure the means by which the process was achieved is fairly clear: for the first time birth control techniques, formerly associated with promiscuity, became an accepted aspect of marital relationships. The decline of the English birth rate dates from 1877 which was the year of the Bradlaugh–Besant trial and there is little doubt that this event, and the publicity which it received, was of great importance in gaining acceptance for the idea, and for the practice, of family limitation.[7] Charles Bradlaugh, already well known as a controversial Member of Parliament, free-thinker and reformer, intervened in the case of a Bristol bookseller who had been found guilty, under the Obscene Publications Act, of selling copies of Knowlton's *Fruits of Philosophy*. There is some doubt whether the edition in question had been enlivened by the inclusion of indelicate illustrations; at any rate Bradlaugh regarded the outcome of the case as a serious challenge to freedom of expression on a subject with which he had long been concerned and, with Mrs Besant, he reprinted the pamphlet and notified the police of his intention to sell it.

Bradlaugh and Mrs Besant were in due course charged, committed, tried, convicted and subsequently acquitted on a technicality during proceedings which lasted over many months and which were fully, often sympathetically, reported in the national and local press. The birth control controversy was thrown 'onto the breakfast-tables of the English middle classes' at a time when, for reasons outlined, they were especially receptive to the message which Bradlaugh and Mrs Besant were attempting to publicize. The judge had made it clear from the outset that he considered the prosecution ill-advised and throughout the course of the trial the defendants and their witnesses made an impressive case for family limitation.[8]

In the meantime, Knowlton's *Fruits of Philosophy*, which before the trial had barely managed to achieve a turnover of a thousand a year, was enjoying a new phase of popularity; during the three months between the arrest of Bradlaugh and the trial 125 thousand copies were sold and a further 60 thousand copies were sold in the period after the trial before being withdrawn as outdated and replaced by a pamphlet by Mrs Besant. For the trial had liberated a new demand for contraceptive knowledge; between 1879 and 1921 more than three million birth control pamphlets and leaflets were circulated, of which at least a third contained detailed contraceptive instruction.[9]

The Bradlaugh–Besant episode had two further consequences for the development of family limitation: the formation of the Malthusian League and the development of a commercial contraceptive trade. The League, which began as a defence fund set up during the trial, persisted as a pressure group and as the forerunner of modern family planning movements. The publicity surrounding the trial and the subsequent activities of the League generated a demand for contraceptive appliances which quickly became the subject of a flourishing, if at times dubious, postal and retail trade. Although, then as now, coitus interruptus was presumably the major method of birth control used, late Victorian parents had a wide range of alternative techniques to choose from. A typical illustrated retail catalogue of 1896 offered the following items:

Rubber Letters—'the best, surest and most frequently used of any known appliance'—in five qualities ranging from 2s. to 10s. per dozen.

Skin Letters—in two sizes ('small and ordinary') and eight qualities (including 'Spanish Curved') ranging from 3s. to 20s. per dozen.

American Tips—at 3s. and 5s. 6d. per dozen.

The 'Rendell' Pessary—soluble quinine pessaries at 2s. per dozen.

The Improved Prolapsus Check Pessaries—in three sizes at 2s. 3d. each.

The Mensinga Pessarie with Spring Rim—in three sizes at 3s. each.

The Gem Pessarie with Sponge Dome—at 5s. each.

The Spring Unique Pessarie with Solid or Inflated Rim—1s. 6d. or 3s. 6d. each.

Inflated Ball Pessaries—in three sizes at 3s. 6d. each.

Contraceptive Sponge—enclosed in silk net 1s. each.

The Combined Pessarie and Sheath—in three sizes at 4s. each.

Quinine Compound—1s. and 2s. per box.

Vulcanite Syringes—at 3s. 6d. each.

Vertical and Reverse Syringes—at 5s. 6d. each.[10]

With the sole exception of the oral contraceptive there is no birth control method in use today which was not available, and available in considerable variety, in the 1890s.

Despite this ready access to contraceptive appliances there is evidence that in late nineteenth-century Britain, as in every other society, abortion had an important role either as an alternative to contraception or as a longstop to contraceptive failure. Precise estimates of the extent of abortion are not available but it would appear that the practice was widespread. In 1898 the Chrimes brothers were sentenced to long terms of penal servitude for blackmailing large numbers of women who had applied to them for abortifacients and it was revealed at the trial that in the course of only three or four days they had obtained £800 in this way. During 1912, in an investigation of family limitation in the north of England, Miss Ethel Elderton noted the widespread practice of self-induced abortion in almost every town and village; pharmacists, herbalists, barbers and market traders, she reported, openly sold abortifacient drugs together with contraceptive appliances.

EXTENT OF CONTRACEPTIVE USAGE

The earliest known attempt to assess the extent of family limitation amongst a sample of the population was a survey conducted by a sub-committee of the Fabian Society in 1905–6 and published by Sidney Webb under the title *The Declining Birth Rate*. The sample consisted of 316 marriages and was drawn from all parts of the country and 'from every section of the middle class'. In answer to the question 'In your marriage have any steps been taken to render it childless or to limit the number of children born?', 242 couples replied 'Yes'. Of the 120 couples who had married between 1890 and 1899 only seven were 'unlimited' and fertile. Webb estimated that, in 1906 one-half, and perhaps two-thirds, of all couples were regulating their families.

In 1946, Lewis-Faning, in a study conducted for the Royal Commission on Population,[11] interviewed, in general wards of selected hospitals, 3,281 women whose first marriage at the time of the survey had not been terminated. These women represented marriages taking place at every decade during the present century and thus provide an illustration of the increasing resort to family limitation for successive cohorts:

Date of marriage	Percentage using contraception at some time during marriage
Before 1910	15
1910–1919	40
1920–1924	58
1925–1929	61
1930–1934	63
1935–1939	66

The low figure for the first group of marriages might appear to contradict the findings of the Fabian survey: the difference, however, is probably wholly accounted for by the contrasting socio-economic groups represented by the two studies and is a confirmation of the fact of differential class usage. For whilst Webb's sample was entirely middle class, Lewis-Faning's women, because of the location of his sample frame, were predominantly of low income and high fertility.

No comparable data relating to the earliest decades of the century are available for the United States but, in commenting on Lewis-Faning's findings, Freedman has suggested[12] that there is no reason to doubt a similar trend. Later American cohorts were even more enthusiastic family planners than their English contemporaries; of the 1,977 white Protestant women who had married during 1927–9 and who were interviewed in the course of the 1941 Indianapolis study 89 per cent had used contraception at some time during marriage.[13]

Investigations based on more recent groups of marriages, in both countries, have shown a continuation of this accelerating resort to birth control and an increase in the proportion of couples who adopt the practice from the outset of marriage rather than at a stage when desired family size has been attained or exceeded. The Population Investigation Committee (PIC) survey in Britain, carried out in 1959, revealed[14] that for those couples married in the 1950s, the percentage ever using contraception had increased to 74 per cent whilst 45 per cent of these couples had begun the practice at marriage, compared with only 36 per cent in the 1930s. A similar tendency is noted in the third report of the Family Growth in Metropolitan America (FGMA) study though precise figures are not given. Amongst couples married in Hull in 1965, 90 per cent were using, had used or intended to use some method of contraception.

PATTERNS OF CONTRACEPTIVE CHOICE

The first detailed and nation-wide survey of the contraceptive practices of married couples was the now classic Indianapolis study of social and psychological factors affecting fertility conducted in 1941. Since then a large number of similar studies in the United States and elsewhere has provided information on patterns of contraceptive choice, on the success rates of different methods and on the influences which tend to govern the choice of method by an individual or by a social group. The most recent comparable national surveys in Britain and America highlight some of the important differences which are to be found in countries of similar social and economic structure and reveal the effect of history and tradition in the overall pattern of choice.

Table 2 compares the pattern of contraceptive usage amongst couples who, in the second Growth of American Families (GAF)[15] study in America and in the PIC study in Britain, had at some time during marriage used birth control techniques. The roughly comparable figures relating to the condom and chemical spermicides reflect the traditional reliance, in both countries, on commercial forms of contraception, the slightly lower figure for the United States representing a lag which no doubt resulted from the years during which, under the Comstock Act, the sale of commercial contraceptives was illegal. When non-appliance

25

TABLE 2. *Comparative popularity of methods in America and Britain 1959*

Contraceptive methods (all users)	British wives married 1930–60	American wives married 1935–55
Percentage reporting use of:		
Condom	49	43
Withdrawal	44	15
Safe period	16	34
Chemicals	16	10
Diaphragm	11	36
Douche	3	28
Other methods	6	4
Total	145	170

methods are considered there are marked differences between the two societies. The high incidence of coitus interruptus in England is in part a result of tradition but also a reflection of a difference in class structure and of continental influences. The corresponding preference for the safe period in the United States may be due to more rigidly held religious convictions; it is also an outcome of a more female-oriented culture which is confirmed by the correspondingly widespread popularity of the douche and the diaphragm. The extent of usage of the latter, in both countries, is a fairly precise index of the extent of medical influence on family planning through the birth control clinic organizations. The over-all average use of 1·7 methods per couple in America, compared with only 1·4 amongst British couples, suggests a greater willingness to experiment with different methods.

Both these surveys were conducted before the oral contraceptive became available and the differential impact of this newest form of birth control further illustrates the different social attitudes in the two countries. The full report of the most recent (1965) GAF study is still awaited but the published figures[16] relating to contraceptive choice show that since its introduction in 1959 the Pill has been used by a third of all American wives and has become the preferred method for a quarter, a situation which might have been predicted on the basis of the established preference for female methods and medically prescribed techniques. In Britain, the oral contraceptive is used by only 16 per cent of married women but here, as elsewhere, there is evidence of an increasing demand for better and more adequate knowledge of family planning techniques.

DIFFERENTIAL FERTILITY

National differences in the overall pattern of contraceptive usage are, in part, the result of historical, including legal and medical, traditions but they are affected too by subcultural influences which determine, in the case of a specific couple, whether birth control will be attempted, what method will be chosen and with what degree of success it will be used. Age, religion, length of education and socio-economic status are merely the most important of a variety of factors which, in numerous studies, have been shown to influence reproductive behaviour.

Family planning minimally involves both a decision on desired family size and the effective limitation of fertility once that size has been reached. In both aspects social factors have been shown to be intervening variables. Exceptionally, these influences may operate in the same direction: Catholic couples, for example, are limited, by the teaching of their church, to a rather ineffective method of birth control but, providentially no doubt, Catholics also show a preference for a larger than average size of family. More usually, however, couples find their contraceptive expertise inadequate to the task which social convention, personal preference and economic necessity impose on them. For most couples the 'problem' of family planning is the problem of not having more children than they want and the degree to which it is resolved varies directly, in advanced societies, with socio-economic status.

Unwanted pregnancies (unwanted, that is, at the time of conception) occur at every social level; the three million pounds annual turnover of the Harley Street abortion industry is sufficient evidence for contraceptive failure in social classes I and II. But the excessively large family, resulting from failure or, more frequently, habitual non-use of contraception is very largely confined to the lower socio-economic groups of all industrial societies. Differential fertility, the social class difference in completed family size, has been a persisting feature of the vital statistics of both Britain and the United States—with the majority of the largest families occurring at precisely those socio-economic levels where, from the point of view of the parents, the existing children and the community, family limitation would be most desirable.

This is the problem area which most clearly justifies medical intervention in the field of family planning; it is perhaps the most neglected, as well as the most potentially rewarding, field of preventive medicine. Children of large families are at a serious disadvantage, physically and socially, in ways which manifest themselves even before birth and which may persist through successive generations of hyperfertility. The chances of fetal wastage and the incidence of infant mortality rise steeply with increasing parity[17] and few doctors can be unaware of the physical ill-health produced by overcrowding and malnutrition or of the high level of maternal morbidity which frequently results from an unimpeded succession of pregnancies.

VOLUNTARY BIRTH CONTROL CLINICS

The early birth control clinics, which were first established in the United States in 1916 and in England in 1921, were intended to provide for precisely this section of the population and the initial clientele of the English clinics appears to have been drawn predominantly from the semi-skilled and unskilled classes IV and V. As figure 2 shows, however, the clinics have not continued to fulfil this function; instead, their clients have come increasingly and disproportionately from the upper-middle and middle classes. In part, this is undoubtedly a reflection of the un-suitability of clinic recommended techniques—caps and diaphragms which, before the availability of the Pill, were virtually the only methods offered—for lower-working-class women. It is also true, however, that women at this socio-economic level have little motivation positively to seek advice by attending a clinic. The prevailing attitude to birth control, as to much else in life, of this section of the population is characterized by Rainwater, in a study entitled *And the Poor Get Children,*[18] as 'doing nothing is the easiest way out'.

One attempt to overcome the problem of hyperfertility has been the establishment of domiciliary birth control schemes which attempt to take the services of the birth control clinic to the home of the working-class family. In a pioneering scheme in Newcastle-upon-Tyne Peberdy[19] demonstrated the undoubted success with which such schemes could be operated. Amongst the first 150 women provided with birth control appliances, the pregnancy rate before entering the project was 130 per hundred woman years (HWY—see p. 45). During the five years of the project the conception rate dropped to 23·7 per HWY; the number of pregnancies thus being reduced to a fifth of the previously prevailing rate.

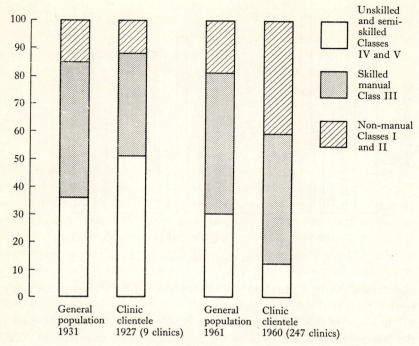

Fig. 2. Class Composition of English clinic patients 1931–61.

THE WORLD POPULATION EXPLOSION

The problem of differential fertility in advanced countries portrays, in microcosm, what on the world scale is implied by the population explosion. For just as large families occur at income levels where they can least be afforded, it is also in those countries which are economically underdeveloped, agriculturally inefficient and low in per capita income that the highest birth rates and the most rapid rate of population growth is taking place. The problem of population growth is now recognized as one of the most urgent issues facing the world. It is a problem which dwarfs all other social, economic and political issues; indeed its very dimensions are such that their implications cannot easily be grasped. Hence the many attempts to present the issue in graphic form: it has taken half-a-million years to produce the existing world population of 3,000,000,000 but at current rates of growth the next 3,000,000,000 will be added in just 35 years; if present rates of population increase were

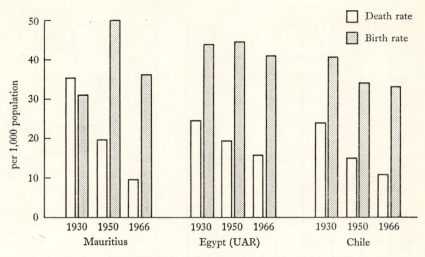

Fig. 3. Selected birth and death rates 1930—1950—1966.

maintained over the next 800 years there would be one person for every square yard of the earth's surface.

The cause of this dramatic situation lies simply in the fact that during the last 25 years death rates in the underdeveloped countries of Asia, Africa and South America, where two-thirds of the world's population lives, have been spectacularly reduced by the adoption of public health programmes and the use of insecticides and antibiotics developed in western countries. One example, from amongst the hundreds which could be cited, illustrates the impact of these developments: malaria, which took three centuries to eradicate in Europe, was eliminated in Ceylon by the use of DDT in less than five years, with an immediate halving of the death rate. Figure 3 shows very clearly, for three other countries, comparable reductions in the mortality rates during the last 30 years.

Figure 3 also shows that this decline in mortality has not been accompanied by a corresponding reduction in the already high birth rates prevailing and with more and more people surviving to become parents the situation very quickly takes on the characteristics of an explosion. The annual rate of world population increase has risen from 1 per cent in 1945 (itself an all-time record) to 1·8 per cent in the mid-1960s. But the differential between the underdeveloped and developed countries, shown in table 3, is seen very clearly to be an outcome of the contrasting pattern

30

TABLE 3. *Percentage increase of world population*

	Birth rate per 1,000	Death rate per 1,000	Annual rate of increase 1960–4 (%)
Developed countries	21	9	1·2
Developing countries	40	20	2·0
World total	34	16	1·8

of births and deaths. The social, economic and political implications of these figures are basic to most of the problems of international relations.

The countries of high population growth are, without exception, those in which the standard of living is already precarious; they are countries characterized by low levels of industrial development and minimal standards of education and personal medical care (the Congo has one practising doctor for every 12,000 inhabitants compared with one per 850 in Britain). They are countries moreover in which growing political awareness and expectations of an improved standard of life give added urgency to the need for a solution to the problem of population growth.

Economic improvement is especially difficult to achieve in a country of high population growth. The age structure of such societies, as illustrated in figure 4, produces a burden of dependency quite unlike that of advanced countries.[20] With large numbers of dependent children requiring expensive education services and correspondingly fewer people in the productive age-groups the problem of increasing the standard of life becomes almost insurmountable. It is nowhere better illustrated than in the United Arab Republic where the High Aswan Dam, an exceptional engineering achievement, is expected to add 40 per cent to the cultivable area of the country. Yet during the time it has taken to plan and build the dam the population has increased by 45 per cent.

A further demographic factor which exacerbates the population problem in many parts of the world is the very low age of marriage of most women. This has the effect both of lengthening the period of exposure to conception, and hence increasing the likely number of pregnancies, and also of foreshortening the length of the generation with a consequent acceleration of geometric growth. In contrast to western Europe where, until recently, age at first marriage remained fairly high,[21] in most of the underdeveloped countries a much larger proportion of girls marry before the age of 20. Consequently whilst the birth rate in England and

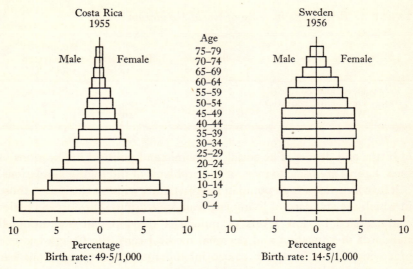

Fig. 4. Population pyramids of developing and developed countries.

Wales even before the adoption of family limitation (see figure 1) never exceeded 35/1,000, in most of the underdeveloped world today the figure is more than 40/1,000 with individual countries showing rates of 45 and 46. In England and the United States there has recently been a fall in the age of women at marriage together with a rise in the birth rate; on the causal connection, as revealed in England and Wales, one demographer has suggested that 'the total extent to which marriages are now occurring at younger ages as compared with before the second world war may have been reflected in an increase of up to 10 per cent in average family size or nearly one quarter of a child per couple'.[22]

The nature of the solution to the world population problem is no longer disputed. It is not to be found in a more equitable distribution of food supplies; already two-thirds of the world's population receives less than the medically recommended dietary intake, and if the whole of the world's food were shared equally we should all be undernourished. Malthus long ago postulated that population, which increases geometrically, will always tend to outstrip food supplies, which can be increased only arithmetically for additional acres of land brought under cultivation. We are now witnessing a startling demonstration of the truth of his thesis. Nor do responsible biologists regard the idea of novelty food supplies (from seaweed, yeast or leaf-protein) as anything more than a remote possibility. The only immediate remedy for the population problem is to counteract death control by positive measures directed to birth control. And just as the former is the outcome of western initiative, in the latter sphere, too, the underdeveloped world has the right to expect guidance from those countries which have already experienced their demographic transition.

Most of the techniques detailed in the following chapters have been used in fertility control programmes in underdeveloped countries; some are obviously more appropriate than others and no method is outstandingly superior for every situation. Nations, like individuals, can be confused and inconsistent in their birth control practices. In Japan, the legalization of abortion in 1949 facilitated a drastic reduction in the birth rate but it was accompanied by a very uneven programme of family planning, and although the government has made some effort to support clinics and to initiate educational effort in contraception, the sale of oral contraceptives is restricted to women with gynaecological indications for their use. The Government of India is now spending £10 million annually on family planning ventures amongst which voluntary male sterilization, with a cash payment to volunteers, appears to be one of the most promising techniques. In Korea and Taiwan the Population Council has, during the past four years, been conducting a programme based on the mass fitting of IUDs; the millionth loop was fitted in Korea in November 1967. Elsewhere the Pill and the condom have been successfully used, although it has been argued that the assumed need for continuing medical supervision of women using the former and the high cost of the latter make these less suitable methods for underdeveloped countries; advances in production technology, research and development are taking place, however, which may lead to these highly effective methods being more widely adopted. The Swedish International Authority is currently supplying several million Pill cycles to Korea and 100,000 gross of condoms to Pakistan each month.

The urgent needs for the future are to extend the range of cheap, acceptable and moderately effective forms of birth control, to make these more widely available and to improve the quality of family planning services. But the problem is not limited to Asia and Latin America— it is a world problem and it is imperative, if it is to be tackled on a global scale, to raise the level of contraceptive practice in the western nations. During the past 150 years it is possible that European and American medical research and clinical practice has been more successful in increasing individual well-being and happiness than has any other communal activity in human history. The single outstanding exception in the potential achievements is that it has failed to provide, and has often opposed, rational methods of lowering the birth rate and of contributing to the universal desire of women to restrict their fertility.

3 THE TESTING AND EVALUATION OF CONTRACEPTIVE METHODS

BACKGROUND

Because the practice of birth control was for so long regarded as being outside the legitimate boundaries of scientific study, the comparative assessment of different contraceptive methods, and even the overall evaluation of family planning practice, is of very recent development. Moreover, the clandestine context of contraceptive sales during the early years of this century was hardly conducive to the development of ethical standards amongst producers and retailers.

There is little doubt that a great deal of worthless rubbish was sold in these early years and as late as 1933 a biochemist reviewing the contemporary trade was able to remark:[1] 'Again and again we find that some product has appeared on the market, has been recalled, reissued (possibly under another name) and the composition changed: the manufacturers appear to be entirely unconcerned about their previous failures and they are emphatic that the new formula will be much more effective...Certain firms do adhere to the standards laid down, do carry out research work, are accurate, honest and truthful in their statements; unfortunately these are in the minority...It is only regrettable that so much real hardship and suffering is permitted through the sale of products so unreliable and so unsatisfactory and which are ultimately purchased by the consumer at such exorbitant prices.'

This undesirable situation had also been commented on in the report of the National Birth Rate Commission which stressed the need for sustained and systematic research and it was with this object in view that the Birth Control Investigation Committee was established in 1927 under the secretaryship of Dr C. P. Blacker of the Eugenics Society. The early activities of the Committee included the statistical analysis of information obtained at birth control clinics, the designing of a standard clinic record card, an enquiry into the contraceptive practices of a sample of the general population, laboratory research on chemical

35

spermicides and rubber appliances and the preparation of a bibliography on spermatoxins.

This programme became a joint Anglo-American endeavour through the collaboration of the US National Committee on Maternal Health which, in the early 1920s and in response to a similar situation in the United States, had drawn up a comprehensive plan for research on chemical contraception. This programme, the Committee had been advised,[2] could not be conducted anywhere in America because the Comstock Act would be invoked against both the publication of research findings and the laboratory synthesis of spermicides. When, in 1929, funds became available for the project the Committee welcomed the opportunity to have the work carried out in Britain in collaboration with the BCIC.

Most of the subsequent advances in the scientific study of contraception have been achieved on the basis of work initiated by these committees, including the development of laboratory techniques for the assay of vaginal contraceptives, the elaboration of statistical formulae for the evaluation of contraceptive efficacy and the development of phenyl mercuric acetate as a spermicide. And whilst in England the BCIC was subsequently responsible for the establishment of the Population Investigation Committee, which publishes the international journal *Population Studies* and which initiated the 1959 survey of contraceptive practice in Britain, the National Committee on Maternal Health was instrumental in the founding of the American Population Council which pioneered the plastic IUD and has been responsible for many other advances in recent years.

THE TESTING OF CHEMICAL SPERMICIDES

The primary requirement of a chemical contraceptive is its capacity to immobilize spermatozoa in human semen. There is a considerable range of laboratory procedures which aim to reproduce in vitro the conditions under which such products act within the vagina; all of them are variants of an original technique devised for the BCIC in 1931 by Baker.[3] They differ principally in that some require the mixing of the semen with the agent under investigation whilst others rely upon diffusion from adjacent deposits of semen and spermicide. Baker's original procedure was of the diffusion type but until recently the preferred method in the United States involved mixing.

Following an extensive review of test procedures the International Planned Parenthood Federation (IPPF) has now proposed[4] a compromise method which involves the partial mixing of semen and spermicide, on the grounds that some co-mingling is produced during coital activity. The test involves few departures from standard laboratory practice and is reproduced in Appendix I of this volume.

The semen used in this, and in any other, test should be obtained by masturbation and collected in a clean glass bottle labelled with donor's name and date and hour of ejaculation and should be used within 4 hours. This may be a serious drawback in laboratories which carry out only occasional tests, but though attempts have been made to use semen obtained from laboratory animals, human semen is much more resistant to most spermicides than that of dogs, rabbits and guinea-pigs. Further investigation in this neglected field of comparative physiology may result in the elaboration of a series of conversion factors which would undoubtedly make the testing of chemical spermicides a more convenient undertaking.

A vaginal contraceptive must of course be non-toxic and non-irritant as well as effectively spermicidal, and the IPPF has published recommended procedures for harmlessness tests on animals and on women. The animal tests include the daily application of the preparation to the vaginae of rhesus monkeys with subsequent assessment by repeated biopsy; an alternative procedure involves the instillation of one-fifth of the human dose into the vaginae of rabbits on fourteen consecutive days followed by gross and microscopic examination for evidence of infection, irritation or epithelial degeneration. Two alternative tests with women are proposed. The '24-hour Cap Test' approved by the Government of India involves, as its name implies, the application of standard doses of the spermicide to the cervices of volunteer women by means of a cervical cap; five volunteers are used for each test and at the end of 24 hours smears are taken for examination using Papanicolaou staining. A procedure developed by the Margaret Sanger Research Bureau relies on twelve volunteers each of whom introduces a single dose of the spermicide deep into the vagina on twenty-one successive nights following the end of menstruation; twice-weekly gynaecological examinations and terminal Papanicolaou smears are undertaken in order to determine the extent of irritation or oedema.

Other irritability tests developed by the Government of India and by the Exeter Family Planning Association in England (misleadingly called 'Acceptability Tests') are based on the reports of randomly selected patients who have agreed to use the product at least once (in the Indian test) or during a period of three months (in the FPA test). In the former case an absence of complaints in at least seventy-five couples out of one hundred is regarded as satisfactory whilst the latter requires an absence of complaints from 90 per cent of the patients. It should be noted, however, that such relative rates will always be to some extent a function of the training and skill of the investigators.

Many contemporary chemical contraceptives rely in part for their effectiveness upon the occlusion of the os by means of the foam produced on dissolution of the product within the vagina. It may thus be necessary to evaluate the foaming capacity of such preparations and this is achieved by adding the standard dose to 4 ml of saline contained in a 100 ml graduated cylinder at 35 to 37 °C. A satisfactory foaming tablet should disintegrate within 2 min to produce 20–40 ml foam, the complete exhaustion of which should require at least 15 min. No test has yet been devised for the evaluation of the physical properties of jellies and pastes, but the Margaret Sanger Research Bureau suggests that suppositories and non-foaming tablets should melt or dissolve without agitation when immersed for 30 min in saline at 37 °C.

THE TESTING OF RUBBER APPLIANCES

Rubber has a long established and still important role in modern contraceptive practice, being used in condoms, caps and diaphragms which in turn are used either alone or in conjunction with chemical spermicides. The properties of these appliances, as well as the effects upon them of storage, lubricants and chemical preparations, are therefore of considerable significance.

1 Condoms

Several organizations, including the Royal Swedish Medical Board, the US Food and Drug Administration and the British Standards Institution have developed tests for rubber condoms all of which are based on variations of the water leakage check. The BSI version of this is reproduced in Appendix II; the FDA procedure is virtually identical except that, instead of examining the suspended condom visually or applying dry filter paper to it, the condom is closed by twisting the neck, and is rolled over an absorbent surface in order to detect any sign of leakage through the walls.

In addition there are recommendations covering quality of manufacturing materials, harmlessness, storage properties, dimensions, weight and labelling. The BSI specification, for example, requires a minimum length of 175 mm (including teat if provided) and a minimum width of 49 mm; it stipulates a maximum allowable weight of 240 g per gross (see chapter 5). A further general requirement is that packages should carry the name or trademark of the manufacturer and the date, including year and month, by which the article is to be used.

The British Standards Specification prescribes an additional 'bursting strength test'—an approximate method of measuring the physical properties of elongation and tensile strength, before and after ageing. This was incorporated in the Standard in place of the more elaborate electronic tensile testing which is expensive and requires highly skilled operators. Deterioration due to storage may be an important hazard with this type of contraceptive method and bursting strength is a useful measure of deterioration. It requires the film to be generally capable of elongation to at least 600 per cent of its original length initially and to retain two-thirds of this value after accelerated ageing for 7 days at 70 °C.—the equivalent of several years of normal shelf life. The bursting strength test may also be used to assess the effects of lubricants or chemical spermicides on rubber and only approved lubricants and spermicidal products should be recommended for use with condoms.

2 Diaphragms

The major potential defects in the vaginal diaphragm are holes and flaws in the membrane, deformation of the spring and separation of the spring joint with subsequent protrusion of the ends through the rim of the device. Visual examination is usually sufficient to reveal imperfections of this type but, because faults are likely to arise during use, patients should be advised to be continually alert for them. Patients should also be taught to compress the spring laterally with fore-finger and thumb and warned that if the spring does not return to its original shape the diaphragm may be ineffective. The British Standards *Specification BS 4028:1966 Diaphragms for Contraceptive Use* makes recommendations on manufacturing materials and the permissible tolerance on sizes and describes an inflation test in which the membrane is inflated to twice its original diameter. Because diaphragms are normally used for periods of up to a year, ageing qualities are especially important and the inflation test must be carried out both before and after accelerated ageing.

3   Cervical and Vault Caps

There are no standard tests for caps other than by visual inspection. The IPPF has suggested that caps may be filled with water and left for 15 min in order to reveal leaks and the English FPA uses a test which involves pushing a round-ended metal rod down the centre of the cap until the dome reaches three times its original size.

THE TESTING OF INTRAUTERINE DEVICES

The testing of IUDs is mainly dependent upon large-scale clinical trials (chapter 10) but some simple checks of the standards of manufacture have been devised. The plastic devices should have a good finish; there should be no variations in colour and the dimensions and weight must conform to the standard specification. The composition of the plastic can be checked by flotations in various concentrations of saline (to ascertain the density) and by incineration when the resulting ash residue should comprise 25 to 30 per cent of the total initial weight. Perhaps the most useful check is the deflection test in which the length of the device is measured before and after elongation for 20 seconds using a 100 g weight—both measurements should be the same.

SCREENING AND PRELIMINARY TRIALS
OF ORAL CONTRACEPTIVES

Toxicity tests and the hormonal activities of any new steroid are conducted on animals. A wide range of properties, including for example glucocorticoid and adrogenic properties, is tested. Separate tests of possible teratogenic activity must also be run.

There are marked species differences in the response to pharmacologically active compounds (Florey said that if penicillin had been tested on guinea-pigs it would have been rejected as too toxic) and nowhere is this more marked than in the field of reproduction. When a new oral contraceptive is tested on a small group of women detailed follow-up of urinary steroids, endometrial biopsies and other physiological parameters can be laid down and the effects on the menstrual cycle evaluated. Trials on 25 patients will permit the optimum dose to be assessed; trials on 100 patients over six months will give some idea of contraceptive effectiveness. Once this stage has been reached further trials will almost certainly be necessary in order to satisfy the requirements of the American Food and Drug Administration and the English Committee on the Safety of Drugs (the Dunlop Committee) and it may take several years before a drug can be marketed.

Statistically, it is much more difficult to deal with an infrequent event, such as one or two pregnancies among 100 women in the course of a year, than it is to compare, for example, two populations for height. The failure rates of oral contraceptives are now so low that it would require records of up to 9 million cycles merely to demonstrate a twofold increase in the effectiveness of a new product. The assessment of the significance of even rarer phenomena, such as embolism, requires very specialized studies on, perhaps, all the women in a nation (see chapter 16).

THEORETICAL EFFECTIVENESS AND
USE-EFFECTIVENESS

Although the theoretical effectiveness of contraceptives, as determined by laboratory tests, may be useful in comparing variants of a particular method (e.g. different chemical compounds as spermicidal agents or different brands of diaphragms and condoms) this can only be a preliminary to more extensive use-effectiveness trials. Indeed, theoretical effectiveness may be quite unrelated to effectiveness in use for a number of reasons. In the first place, laboratory tests can never adequately replicate the in vivo circumstances in which a contraceptive may be used. Thus, in the now well-known tests of chemical spermicides carried out by Masters & Johnson[5] using the technique of artificial coitus, the cream which achieved the highest rating was also the most spermicidal on mixing tests but was inefficient on diffusion tests; on the other hand the most efficient jelly in the artificial coitus test had a low rating on mixing tests but was highly spermicidal on diffusion tests.

Secondly, physiological and behavioural idiosyncracies may operate to modify the efficacy of a particular method. The theoretical effectiveness of the 'safe period', for example, can be evaluated statistically by techniques of considerable sophistication and accuracy. In practice, however, the method is far less reliable than the calculations suggest because of the unpredictability of the menstrual cycle in most women and in particular its susceptibility to the effects of concurrent illness. Again artificial coitus has been used to demonstrate that the effectiveness of the vaginal diaphragm is very much dependent upon the coital position or alternation of positions adopted by the users, its maximum efficiency being achieved only in the male superior position.

The third and most important factor which operates to modify the theoretical efficacy of a contraceptive method is represented by a complex of social and psychological variables which are collectively summarized in the concept of 'acceptability'. Thus, a method which may have high theoretical efficiency, such as total or partial abstinence, may be ineffective for most couples because of its low acceptability. Conversely relatively inefficient, even irrational, methods may survive because they are found to be acceptable. Acceptability involves a wide range of factors amongst which the extremes are represented by individual psychological motivations on the one hand and broad regional or ethnic influences on the other. Within a particular society, however, the most important components are those subcultural influences, including education, socio-economic status, age and income, which affect the care, perseverance and consequent success with which a particular method is used.

For a specific couple, moreover, the acceptability of a given method may depend upon the precise stage in the family building process at which it is adopted, in particular upon whether it is being used to delay a pregnancy in an incompleted family or to prevent any further pregnancy in a family already regarded as adequate. One of the most significant findings of the second Family Growth in Metropolitan America (FGMA)[6] study was the marked improvement in the efficiency of contraceptive usage as couples approached the number of children desired.* Table 4 (which is adapted from that study) shows that efficiency was also related to the size of desired family but whatever the total number of children contemplated contraception improves with increasing parity.

TABLE 4. *Contraceptive failure rates (per hundred women years) in each of three intervals for couples using traditional methods*

	No. of children desired			
Interval	2	3	4 or more	Total
Marriage to first pregnancy	21	27	46	30
First to second pregnancy	8	14	16	12
Since second live birth	3	16	13	9
All intervals	10	19	24	16

There is also a tendency for couples to adopt more efficient techniques as their families grow and theoretical effectiveness and acceptability may become interacting factors especially in a society where the relative merits of contraceptive techniques are publicly discussed; they will, however, never precisely coincide. It is for this reason that an adequate evaluation of a contraceptive technique must be based on the actual reproductive behaviour of a representative group of couples known to be using that particular method.

USE-EFFECTIVENESS OF CONTRACEPTIVE METHODS

Before the establishment of birth control clinics, and in the absence of extensive social surveys, it was impossible to carry out statistical studies either on selected groups of users or amongst representative sections of the general population. Unfortunately the first birth control clinics were more anxious to use the new evidence and opportunities created by their work as a justification for their own preferred choice of technique rather than to attempt any objective appraisal of alternative

* The term 'suffiparous' would appear to be a useful designation for women of this type.

methods. Thus Marie Stopes claimed[7] a 99·4 per cent success rate for her cervical cap but imputed an 85·5 per cent *failure* rate to the diaphragm recommended by the 'rival' clinics of the Society for the Provision of Birth Control Clinics (now the FPA). In reply, Dr Norman Haire, medical officer of the SPBCC Walworth Clinic, claimed that the diaphragm was far superior to the Stopes cap which had, he declared,[8] failed in 88 per cent of all those cases which he had seen.

What both Marie Stopes and Norman Haire were in complete agreement on was the almost total unreliability of every method of birth control other than those recommended by their respective organizations. Patients coming to them for advice were questioned about previous methods used and from this data, comprising 1,284 Stopes' cases and 1,800 SPBCC patients, the following failure rates were calculated:

	Percentage of failures reported by	
Pre-clinic method	Haire	Stopes
Condom	51·1	75·3
Douche	73·5	95·1
Caps	87·5	—
Diaphragms	—	85·5
Quinine suppositories	70·8	98·1
Withdrawal	69·5	81·8
Safe period	100·0	100·0

In both sets of data failures were taken to include all unwanted pregnancies which had occurred during the use of a particular method taking into account neither how long that method had been used nor with what degree of care. Conversely, the success rates claimed for clinic-recommended methods related to all those patients who had been supplied with caps or diaphragms but who had not returned to report a pregnancy! Marie Stopes defended this novel statistical procedure on the grounds that persons with a grievance are noisy and used the supporting analogy that 'in one's own life one complains if the milk is sour but says no word of praise or thanks to the milkman who daily delivers fresh milk'.

These comparisons of clinic and pre-clinic contraceptive experiences were further biased in favour of the clinic techniques by two additional factors which both Stopes and Haire chose to ignore. The first was the essentially self-selecting nature of the clinic clientele. For every woman who came to the clinics because of dissatisfaction with traditional methods there were obviously many hundreds of others who continued to use those methods with relative success; the clinics' patients were thus not merely biased against traditional methods, they were also more highly motivated to the conscientious use of the appliances provided by the clinics. The second factor was the failure to standardize the length of experience relating to different methods; in virtually every case the clinic experience used in the calculation was of shorter duration than the pre-clinic experience and therefore less likely to reveal a representative failure rate.

But despite these many shortcomings the early pioneers of birth control had laid the basis for a more systematic study of contraceptive efficacy, and subsequent developments in the statistical appraisal of methods and techniques are most readily understood as progressive attempts to overcome the inadequacies of these earlier assessments. In particular, their exclusive concentration on effectiveness in use rather than on theoretical or laboratory effectiveness was a perfectly justifiable procedure and it is now universally accepted that any comparative evaluation of contraceptive methods must be based on use-effectiveness, that is, the degree to which such methods are successfully used by couples enjoying regular coitus to reduce the incidence of unwanted pregnancies.

DETERMINATION OF USE-EFFECTIVENESS

The use-effectiveness of a contraceptive method is defined in terms of its capacity to prevent unwanted pregnancies. It is usually expressed in terms of a failure rate per hundred woman years of exposure and abbreviated as HWY. The basis for calculating this failure rate is known as Pearl's Formula[9] which is expressed:

$$\text{Failure rate per HWY} = \frac{\text{Total accidental pregnancies} \times 1,200.}{\text{Total months of exposure}}$$

In any application of this formula the total accidental pregnancies shown in the numerator must include every known conception whatever its outcome; the factor 1,200 is, of course, the number of months in 100 years. The total months of exposure in the denominator is obtained by deducting from the period under review all those months during which, for extrinsic reasons, conception was not possible; by convention ten months is deducted for a full-term pregnancy and four months for an abortion.

The standardization achieved by this index can be thought of as the number of unwanted pregnancies which would occur either amongst 100 women using a particular technique for one year or to a hypothetical woman experiencing a century of fecundity and coital activity. There is much evidence that, in the complete absence of birth control practice, the pregnancy rate would be about 40, a figure which seems relatively constant from society to society and amongst different socio-economic groups.[10] This corresponds to a total of about 10 to 12 children during an average reproductive lifetime and the notion of failure rates per HWY is perhaps more meaningful to a lay enquirer if it is interpreted as four times the number of accidental pregnancies which would occur during 25 years of marriage.

Our knowledge of contraceptive failure rates derives from two major sources: demographic studies and clinical trials. The former are usually concerned with representative samples of particular populations and include the full range of methods currently in use. Clinical studies, on the other hand, usually include only volunteer (and to this extent atypical) couples and are confined to specific, usually clinic-recommended, methods. Whilst demographic studies are retrospective and thus subject to error through faulty recall, clinical trials are concurrent or prospective and, however adequately supervised, are subject to loss through failure to retrace every patient.

It is with this latter type of study that doctors are most likely to be personally concerned and a number of important points should be observed in designing and interpreting a use-effectiveness trial. A minimum of 600 months of exposure is usually considered necessary[11] before any firm conclusion can be reached and it is important that this should represent an adequate compromise between a large sample with short exposure (and the consequent over-representation of short-term side effects) and a small sample with lengthier exposure (and the danger of loss through other factors). Higher failure rates are invariably recorded in the early months of use-effectiveness trials because careless usage is quickly exposed and is self-eliminating. It is also essential that couples taking part in any trial should be as representative as possible, especially of the different stages of family building. Social class, length of education and age are also important factors in determining contraceptive success.

The deduction, from months of exposure, of those periods when conception was impossible, is a matter of basic experimental design. What

46

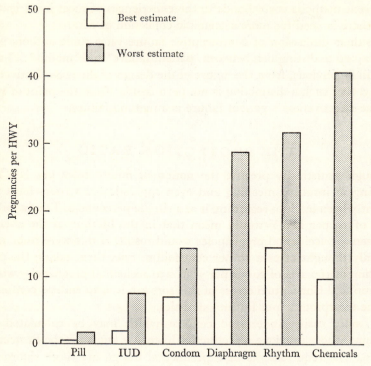

Fig. 5. Failure rates of contraceptive methods.

appears to have been overlooked in all evaluations of the rhythm method is the fact that abstinence is demanded of couples using this method during at least a third of the cycle and often for as much as half (see chapter 8). Strictly, therefore, the period of exposure should be reduced accordingly and the published failure rates for this method are obviously grossly overstated. These methodological points as well as the essential differences between clinical trials and demographic surveys should be kept in mind in interpreting tables which attempt to compare different methods; indeed, the validity of presenting data in this way is highly questionable. The experience of Puerto Rican recruits to a demographic study in 1942 is not comparable with that of self-selected clients of a Baltimore family planning clinic in 1965 and it is misleading to present the two sets of data in this way. For this reason figure 5 has been constructed to show best and worst estimates derived from studies which the authors regard as broadly analogous. The resulting rank order of different methods corresponds to the experiences of most investigators but there is need for more systematic collection of data.

In their discussion of contraceptive failure rates some authors have attempted to distinguish between 'patient failure' and 'method failure'. It will be obvious, from the nature of the design of the use-effectiveness study, that such a distinction is not permissible; from the point of view of use-effectiveness a patient failure is a method failure.

THE PROTECTION RATIO

Though statistically precise, the notion of failure rates per HWY is lacking in intuitive meaning and even sophisticated writers have frequently been led into regarding it as a simple percentage. Thus a failure rate of 10 per HWY would mean that in the lifetime of the average woman 2·5 accidental pregnancies would result. If this were to be mistakenly thought of as a 10 per cent failure rate, then, taking the convention of 100 acts of coitus per year, 250 accidental pregnancies would be implied! Conceptual errors of this sort can lead to endless confusion in the interpretation of fertility statistics.

A more easily understood concept which may be calculated for patients whose previous reproductive history is known is the Protection Ratio. The requirements of experimental design are more rigorously fulfilled in this calculation since the previous unprotected experience of the couples participating provides a control. Thus, in a domiciliary birth control project conducted in Newcastle-upon-Tyne, Peberdy[12] found that the conception rate of her couples in the years of marriage up to the time of entering the scheme was 130·2 per HWY (these couples had been specifically selected for hyperfertility and thus considerably exceeded the general average of 80 per HWY). During the five years of the survey the conception rate dropped to 23·7 per HWY and the protection ratio was thus

$$\frac{(130\cdot2 - 23\cdot7)}{130\cdot2} \times 100 = 81\cdot5.$$

4 COITUS INTERRUPTUS

HISTORY AND EXTENT OF USAGE

Coitus interruptus is an ancient, probably the earliest, form of birth control practice. It is well known in most parts of the world under a variety of names and euphemisms which, although they reflect its widespread usage, may in specific enquiries have tended to obscure the extent of its popularity. Whilst 'withdrawal', 'coitus incompletus' and 'being careful' are virtually international terms, local idioms such as 'getting off at Cottingham instead of going through to Beverley' (a term used in Hull but having many regional equivalents) are likely to mislead survey interviewers unless they have been adequately briefed.

In eighteenth- and nineteenth-century Europe coitus interruptus played an important part in the demographic transition[1] and has remained a major method of contraception. In a study of 3,300 marriages carried out for the Royal Commission on Population in England in 1947 it was found[2] that amongst recently married couples with contraceptive experience 43 per cent had used withdrawal as a sole method of birth control, the proportion rising to 61 per cent amongst couples in Social Class V. Ten years later the PIC survey revealed[3] that 20 per cent of couples had never tried any other method and a further 19 per cent had reverted to it after attempting to use some other technique. The social class gradient persisted but even amongst non-manual groups withdrawal was the preferred method for a fifth of all couples.

Withdrawal is less popular in the United States where, according to recent surveys, fewer than 5 per cent of couples have adopted it as their sole method although 18 per cent have used it on occasions.[4] These figures are indicative of a relatively recent shift in the pattern of contraceptive practice, however, since an analysis[5] of twelve enquiries conducted between 1917 and 1934 and covering 25,000 couples showed that two-thirds of these admitted to having used withdrawal. Studies in many other societies have also revealed extensive usage: by 60 per cent of couples in Jamaica,[6] 54 per cent in Puerto Rico and 67 per cent in Hungary.[7] In India there appears to be a reversal of the social class gradient noted in western countries: whilst only 25 per cent of couples in a village study relied on the method,[8] it was used by 42 per cent of a sample of medical doctors in Uttar Pradesh and by 45 per cent upper-class Hindu families in Calcutta.[9]

Such a universal and widespread usage is obviously a reflection of high acceptability and this is further supported by evidence that, for many couples, withdrawal is a *preferred* method. A study[10] of 750 non-persisting patients from the Birmingham FPA clinic in 1959 showed that 91 per cent had changed from the diaphragm to some other method and that of these 58 per cent had chosen coitus interruptus. Although herself opposed to the method the investigator commented: 'Dependence on coitus interruptus is so widespread that many women think of it not as a contraceptive but rather as a normal part of sexual intercourse. In a number of instances the husband had become so accustomed to withdrawing that he was unable to give up the practice when the wife wore a cap.'

RELIABILITY

Testimony of this kind stands in sharp contrast to the aesthetic biases which most middle-class commentators have revealed in discussing coitus interruptus. All too often, too, this bias has encouraged condemnation of the practice not merely on hygienic grounds but also on grounds of reliability and psychological hazards. The high failure rates alleged by the early clinic personnel have been noted (p. 44) and these have been quoted and re-quoted by two generations of writers with the result that withdrawal has become synonymous with ineffective contraceptive usage. Yet the evidence contradicts this view. As long ago as 1949 the Royal Commission on Population reported[11] that 'no difference has been found between users of appliances and users of non-appliance methods as regards the average number of children'. Amongst those relying on non-appliance methods of all kinds (of which withdrawal was, of course, the most popular) the pregnancy rate was 8 per 100 years of exposure. In the Princeton study the overall pregnancy rate for those couples practising withdrawal was 17 per HWY compared with 14 for the condom and diaphragm and 38 for the 'safe period'.[12] The Indianapolis study revealed[13] a failure rate of only 10 compared with an average rate of 12 for all other methods, and amongst high-income couples the rate was 3, precisely the same figure as for the diaphragm. In Calcutta an extensive survey revealed that pregnancy rates were lower at each occupational level for those employing withdrawal than for those using traditional methods.[14]

SAFETY

It has recently become less fashionable to condemn coitus interruptus as a physically and psychologically injurious technique. In the past a variety of disturbances have been attributed to its use including prostatic hypertrophy and impotence in men and pelvic congestion and frigidity in women. There are no reliable data to suggest a causal relationship between method and symptoms. On the other hand there is some evidence that the use of the method, especially where it is insisted upon by one partner despite the explicit objections or wishes of the other, may lead to tension and a consequent deterioration of sexual relationships.

EVALUATION AND CLINICAL CONSIDERATIONS

Requiring neither prior preparation nor medical supervision and costing nothing, coitus interruptus is widely practised without apparent harm and with considerable success. If there are no good reasons for recommending it neither are there any obvious grounds for discouraging it among couples who have already decided on the method and appear to be relatively happy with it. An official Indian family planning manual,[15] which in its earlier editions condemned the practice, now advises: 'It is condemned by some doctors, but try it. You won't suddenly become a nervous wreck. If you notice bad effects you can easily give it up.' This seems to be as much and as little as the medical adviser will need to say.

5 THE CONDOM

HISTORICAL

In Britain, and indeed throughout the world, the condom is the most widely used birth control device; it is also one of the oldest. In the folklore of contraception its invention is attributed to a Dr Condom who was reputedly a physician at the court of Charles II. The story, as commonly related,[1] suggests that the king, who had become alarmed at the numbers of his illegitimate offspring, subsequently knighted the doctor in recognition of this unique contribution to monarchical welfare.

It is certain, however, that the device was well known before the reign of Charles II (1660–85) and it is doubtful whether any such person as Condom ever existed. More probably the term which first appeared in print in 1717 as 'condum', was derived from the Latin (condus: a receptacle) as a euphemism for an article already widely known. There are, indeed, a score of terms by which the device has been known at various times, and it is significant that whilst the French refer to it as 'la capote anglaise' we have reciprocated with the term 'french letter', 'letter' being a fairly recent corruption of the word 'envelope'.

The earliest published description of the condom is that of the Italian physician Fallopio who, in 1564, recommended a linen sheath, moistened with a lotion, to be used as a protection against venereal infection. In 1597 Hercule Saxonia described a similar device made from some kind of fabric soaked in a solution of inorganic salts and subsequently allowed to dry. The condom was still regarded primarily as a prophylactic a century later when Mme Sevigne, in a much-quoted letter to her daughter the Comtesse de Grignan, describes a sheath made from gold-beaters' skin as 'armour against love, gossamer against infection'.

By the eighteenth century the condom 'preservative', 'machine', or 'armour', as it was variously described, had achieved some popularity for its contraceptive as well as its prophylactic function and it was widely praised in the erotic poetry of the period. In his *London Journal* Boswell tells how, on 10th May, 1763, he 'picked up a strong young jolly damsel, led her to Westminster Bridge and there, in armour complete, did I enjoy her upon this noble edifice'.[2] From the mid-eighteenth century there is evidence of a flourishing trade in London largely in the hands of Mrs Perkins and Mrs Philips whose advertisements gained a wide circulation and contained the invitation:

> 'To guard yourself from shame or fear,
> Votaries to Venus hasten here,
> None in my ware e'er found a flaw,
> Self-preservation's nature's law.'

Mrs Philips, in a handbill dated 1796,[3] boasted 35 years' experience and claimed to supply 'apothecaries, chemists and druggists' as well as 'ambassadors, foreigners, gentlemen and captains of ships going abroad' with 'any quantity of the best goods in England on the shortest notice and at the lowest price'.

The condoms of this period were apparently made from the caeca of sheep or other animals and there is an illustration, in a publication of 1744,[4] which shows men and women seated at a table engaged in their manufacture. In 1952 a locked box was discovered in the muniment room of an English country mansion and when opened it was found to contain a quantity of these early condoms in three different sizes, double-wrapped in packets of eight. One of these was examined by Dingwall of the British Museum who was able to date it between 1790 and 1810 and who described it as 'being made of some animal membrane and, as far as could be discovered, seamless, the edge of the open end being turned over and roughly stitched with cotton to form a hem through which is threaded a strip of silk. Its approximate dimensions are: length 190 mm, diameter 60 mm, thickness 0·038 mm.'[5]

These early skin condoms were expensive and obviously beyond the means of the growing number of couples who, during the latter part of the nineteenth century, were beginning to practise family limitation. It was fortuitous, therefore, that the vulcanization of rubber, first carried out by Hancock and Goodyear in 1844, could be applied to the manufacture of condoms, and from the 1870s this device entered a new phase of popularity.

METHODS OF MANUFACTURE

If the vulcanization of rubber revolutionized the world's transport, its impact on sexual relations and the family building habits of western society has been no less significant. The replacement of the skin sheath by the rubber condom in the late nineteenth century, made available an inexpensive, hygienic and reliable method of contraception at the precise time when family limitation was beginning to be regarded as an essential aspect of married life, and the condom figures very prominently in the contraceptive catalogues of the 1890s.

The earliest rubber condoms were moulded from sheet crepe and although a satisfactory standard of subsequent vulcanization could be achieved the finished product carried a seam along its entire length. By the end of the nineteenth century, however, this defect had been overcome and seamless 'cement' process condoms were being produced by dipping hollow glass formers into a solution of crepe rubber in petroleum solvent, the resulting film being vulcanized by exposure to sulphur dioxide. The earliest teat-ended products, which appeared in the literature in 1901 under the trade-name 'Dreadnought', were made by this process.

The major technological improvement however was the development, in the early 1930s, of the latex process. Glass formers were dipped directly into liquid latex (the sap of the rubber tree suspended in water and stabilized with ammonia and anti-oxidants) and curing was achieved by re-dipping the formers, now covered with a thin film of latex, into hot water. The resulting product had an infinitely better appearance, could be stored for five years instead of three months and had double the tensile strength of the 'cement' article.[6]

The rapid expansion of both domestic and world markets during the last 40 years has stimulated further refinements in the basic latex process, particularly the mechanization and automation of the manufacturing equipment which facilitate the production of a more uniform quality of article. The highly automated plant, which is now used by the major manufacturers in Britain and in the United States, consists of a 400 feet long conveyor moving successively, at the rate of 40 feet per minute, over latex tanks, heated air chambers, hot water baths and sets of roller-brushes. On each side of the conveyor are suspended glass formers 35 cm (14 in) long and 4 cm (1½ in) in diameter which are continuously rotated during their passage through the system. They first enter the liquid latex at an angle of 45° and, after gathering a film, are brought out at an elevation which is designed to impart a slight thickening to the rubber at the tip of the product. After passing through a drier they are re-dipped in order to produce a laminated condom with a total thickness of 0·05 ±0·01 mm. The open end is beaded on the former by passage through a set of brushes which roll down the still liquid latex prior to passage, for vulcanization, through heated air chambers. After further drying the finished product is rolled, by means of nylon brushes, off the former which is then cleansed before re-entering the latex on its next circuit.

Such automatic plants are operated, with a minimum of manual supervision, during 24 hours of the day and, except for brief periods of maintenance, continuously throughout the year. The flow, viscosity, and pH of the latex are automatically controlled, as are the temperature and humidity of the drying and curing chambers. At full production, plants of this type are capable of producing half a million gross of condoms per year. Total annual production in the UK is approximately 200 million of which about half are exported. The Swedish International Development Authority is currently supplying 170 million condoms to Pakistan each year.

A further important innovation has been the recent introduction of the pre-lubricated condom. The idea of pre-lubrication is by no means new: for many years United States manufacturers have marketed condoms in sealed capsules containing glycerine or glycol. The development of a semi-dry lubricated product in 1960, however, resulted from the application of the ubiquitous silicones to the final packaging, 0·30 g of a specially developed product being simply injected into the centre of the rolled condom prior to sealing and allowed to migrate over the whole surface of the article during storage. These are the so-called 'gossamer' products which are said to give increased sensitivity in use. At any rate, since their introduction some eight years ago their share of total domestic sales in England has risen to 85 per cent.

QUALITY CONTROL

It appears to have been the practice of manufacturers, from the earliest days, to apply some sort of testing procedure to their products and in the first decades of the present century the more reputable firms carried out inflation tests on each item before despatch. In 1951 automated machinery was adapted to the electronic testing of each individual condom in what is virtually an extension of the production process. This routine is based on the fact that rubber is a poor conductor of electricity and the condoms are drawn, by hand, on to a second series of moving formers, in this case of metal and large enough to distend the condom under test. The loaded formers are then immersed in water contained in a metal tank and when both tank and former are electrically charged pinholes and even weak patches in the rubber are detected, defective items being automatically removed from the production line for destruction. This process is virtually as costly as the actual manufacture but, together with sample tests carried out at subsequent stages of handling and packaging, it ensures conformity to standards of reliability which are now incorporated in the import regulations of many foreign governments and which have recently been formalized in a British Standard Specification.

THE BSI SPECIFICATION FOR RUBBER CONDOMS

Following discussions with the Family Planning Association and with the manufacturers the British Standards Institution published, in March 1964,[7] the first British specification for contraceptives. The standards outlined cover such comprehensive requirements as quality of manufacturing materials, harmlessness of the product, freedom from defects, strength, storage properties, dimensions, weight and labelling.

Manufacturers licensed to use the BSI's seal of approval (the well-known 'Kitemark') are obliged to conduct quanta tests on each production batch. The number of test specimens taken in the course of manufacture is based on a formula which is calculated so as to accept up to 0·5 per cent of defective items in production batches made under approved manufacturing conditions. In addition the Institute has the right to ensure the conformity of the products of its licensees by testing samples taken from the manufacturers' works, stores and warehouses and from points of sale in the open market. Condoms marketed by licensed manufacturers must carry, in addition to the BSI reference number, the name or trademark of the manufacturer and the date, including year and month, by which the article is to be used. Denmark, Sweden, Japan and the US have somewhat similar standards.

EXTENT OF CONTEMPORARY USAGE

The condom has been, and remains, the most widely used contraceptive device in Britain and in other western societies. Amongst the 1,340 couples married in the period 1930–49 who were interviewed in the course of the PIC study in 1959 (see chapter 2) 48 per cent had used condoms at some time during marriage and 36 per cent were current users. Similarly, in the Family Growth in Metropolitan America study in 1957, 31 per cent of the 1,165 white couples interviewed were using the condom as the sole method of birth control and a further 10 to 15 per cent were using the condom in combination with some other method. In Japan consecutive nationwide surveys have shown an increase in the use of the condom from 38 per cent of the general population in 1950 to 58 per cent in 1959.[8]

The PIC study revealed a greater reliance on the condom amongst younger couples and, in the 1950 cohort of marriages, an increasing usage with rising social status. Thus, whilst the percentage of condom users in the unskilled and semi-skilled manual grades was 29, in the skilled manual grades it was 34 and in non-manual white-collar and professional grades 39. On the other hand, there is evidence from domiciliary birth control schemes that the condom has a high acceptance rate amongst low income groups.[9] A satisfactory acceptance rate for the condom has also been inferred both from the Indianapolis Study in which the proportion of couples changing their contraceptive practice was lower for the condom than for any other method, and from the PIC study which revealed that four out of every five condom users had never tried any other method.

These surveys were, of course, carried out before the oral contraceptive became widely available. But whilst it appears that in the United States condom usage has declined as more and more women have begun to use the Pill, in Britain oral contraceptors appear to have been recruited largely from those who previously used chemical spermicides or non-appliance techniques. The Hull Marriage Survey showed no decline in condom usage amongst couples married in 1965 compared with the earlier marriages investigated in the PIC survey and an independent retail survey carried out nationally in the same year suggested[10] that the widespread publicity which the Pill and the IUD has attracted had also benefited sales of traditional products whilst non-appliance methods had declined in popularity.

TYPES AVAILABLE

Although condoms are commercially available under more than sixty different trade names, in a variety of colours and packs and at widely varying prices, most of the 100 millions sold annually in Britain are of latex variety and amongst these the pre-lubricated product is the most popular. Condoms are invariably rolled and hermetically sealed in aluminium foil sachets; they are retailed in packs of three, the major outlets being men's hairdressers and pharmacies, which together account for approximately 63 per cent of the trade, mail order and surgical stores accounting for 20 per cent. The balance is supplied by miscellaneous outlets such as factory sales, vending machines and FPA clinics. Most of the condoms sold in Britain are teat-ended but this is an essentially national idiosyncracy and consumers in the rest of Europe and in the U.S. universally prefer the plain-ended variety. Some manufacturers, particularly in Germany and Japan, produce coloured condoms; black and red are both popular.

A few washable sheaths are still sold; these are manufactured from thicker latex and are intended for repeated use. There is, in fact, no reason why a good quality disposable condom should not be used more than once provided that it is carefully washed, dried and re-rolled; all this requires the greatest care and is, of course, impossible when lubricated products are used. For most couples it would appear to be hardly worth the time and trouble involved.

A variety of condom which appears in many surgical stores and mail order advertisements, and which must be strongly condemned, is the American or Grecian tip. This is a short condom, with a tightly constricted bead, which covers only the glans of the penis, thus producing, according to the advertisers, less interference and desensitization. The glans is, of course, the most sensitive part of the penis and such a device would appear to be unnecessary as well as unsafe.

A recent innovation in the condom market has been the re-introduction of skin condoms, in the form of lamb caeca. These are individually encapsulated in glycol and are claimed to be superior to the latex product by assuring greater sensitivity, the animal membrane being a better conductor of heat than rubber and the device more loosely fitting over the major part of its length. At three to four times the price of the best quality latex product they are clearly intended as luxury items.

Condoms are sold under a variety of trade names from 'Abdullah' to '777' and including such amphibologues as 'Gold Carriage', 'Patrician', 'Waverley Pearl' and 'Ramses'.

CLINICAL ASPECTS

The major virtue of the condom, of course, is precisely that it is easily obtainable from non-clinical sources and can be used without medical supervision. Its persisting popularity undoubtedly derives from the fact that it can be bought without prescription and if necessary from sources other than pharmacies. Indeed, for individuals wishing to pursue their sex lives in complete privacy (and even in swinging Britain there must be a few introvert souls) the vending machine represents the ideal medium through which an impersonal purchase may be made.

Nevertheless there is a limited range of cases in which specific clinical indications for the use of the condom exist. These include cases of vaginal trichomoniasis and moniliasis where there is a likelihood of re-infestation by the male; cases in which the anatomical condition of the female precludes the fitting of a diaphragm; cases in which it is psychologically necessary that the male should retain control of reproduction; cases of premature ejaculation in which the condom may be effective in prolonging coitus and cases in which immediate reassurance of successful protection against conception is psychologically important to one or both partners.

In addition to this group of cases the condom can also be recommended as a reliable and harmless method of contraception, particularly as an interim method or as an alternating technique for couples who wish to share the responsibility for birth control. It is the ideal method of contraception for couples whose acts of intercourse are sporadic or unpredictable. There is little point in prescribing the oral contraceptive for a wife who is likely to see her seafaring husband only twice a year; the condom would appear to be both more satisfactory and less expensive. Similarly, the unmarried, for whom intercourse may be isolated and spontaneous, will usually find the condom a satisfactory receptacle for wild oats.

The condom is the one form of contraception which is virtually without clinical contraindications or side effects of any kind; a thorough search of the literature of the last 30 years has revealed only one reported case of alleged side effects.[11]

Family planning organizations, because of their exclusively female orientation, have tended to under-rate the condom. But, because of its high acceptability and effectiveness doctors should be reluctant to discourage its use amongst couples who have used it successfully for a number of years.

USE AND CARE

Although, because of its simplicity, the condom is less open to misuse than most other forms of contraception its efficacy can be enhanced by clinical instruction and, since most failures result from carelessness in use rather than from defects in the product, professional interest and intervention is undoubtedly justified.

Modern methods of manufacture and testing have obviated the need for any individual re-testing before use; indeed, attempts to inflate by blowing may merely result in damage to the article through contact with a jagged finger-nail. Nor is it essential, despite the repeated statements which have been made to the contrary, that the condom should be worn during foreplay and initial penetration. The sperm-count of pre-ejaculatory secretions is far lower than in normal ejaculates and the risk of conception is minimal.[12] In most males its occurrence is, in any case, irregular.[13] On the other hand it is essential that the condom is placed in position well before ejaculation takes place and that it is worn correctly.

The condom should be unrolled onto the erect penis, care being taken that the air is expelled from the teat or, in the case of a plain-ended article, that a portion of the closed end is deflated and left free. If this precaution is omitted the occluded air may either rupture the condom or more probably may be forced towards, and overflow from the open end. For the same reason withdrawal should be carefully undertaken with the open end firmly held to ensure that the condom does not slip off, especially if detumescence has occurred.

In those cases where a contraceptive failure would be disastrous the condom should be used in conjunction with an approved spermicide in either pessary or paste form. This reduces the risk of pregnancy if a mechanical failure should occur and also assists in lubrication. It is, of course, essential that the condom should be used on every occasion and the, not uncommon, alternation of condom and safe period (the latter usually being calculated carelessly or erroneously) is a practice which should be discouraged.

EVALUATION

Traditionally outside the sphere of clinical concern, the condom has usually been regarded as a 'merely commercial' and therefore—by some perverse logic—unreliable form of contraception. Certainly those women who have presented themselves at birth control clinics have often alleged earlier condom failures. However, clinical history-taking within establishments manifestly offering other forms of contraception and from clearly self-selected patients is hardly a substitute for controlled trials and their experience stands in sharp contrast to the general popularity of the device amongst the wider population.

When, during the 1950s, more reliable and representative data became available from the first retrospective studies of wider sections of the population it became clear that the condom had a remarkably high rate of use-effectiveness. Commenting on the Family Growth in Metropolitan American findings, Tietze concluded[14] that a group of normally fecund couples copulating 120 times per year and carefully using a good grade of condom on every occasion would experience an accidental pregnancy rate of about 3 per 100 years of exposure. This estimate appears to be confirmed by the limited number of controlled trials which have been carried out in Britain and from which it is possible to make the necessary calculations.

International family planning programmes, like the birth control clinics of advanced societies, have for long ignored the condom as a viable method of fertility control. But the Population Council (which began the research in 1959 which was eventually responsible for the rehabilitation of the IUD after years of neglect) has very recently[15] begun to sponsor the manufacture of plastic condoms. These are stamped from ethylene ethyl acrylate sheets. Like disposable gloves they are made in two pieces, heat sealed together (though the seam is virtually imperceptible) and with a rubber ring sealed within the open end. They differ from the latex product in being thinner (0·025 mm), in having unlimited storage life, greater lubricity, and a more appropriate shape (based on the contour of the caecal condom).

Plastic condoms are manufactured by simple and inexpensive equipment which can be installed in underdeveloped countries and operated by unskilled indigenous workers. Annual production, from a plant costing £3,000 and operating continuously throughout the year is estimated at 10,000 gross. It is just conceivable that the very appliance which has contributed so fully to the demographic revolution in western societies may, in its new form, provide an important part of the answer to the world population explosion.

6 DIAPHRAGMS AND CERVICAL CAPS

HISTORICAL

Given even an elementary knowledge of the physiology of reproduction the occlusion of the cervix appears as an obvious and persisting method of contraception. There is a vast literature relating to historical and pre-literate societies in which a variety of gums, leaves, fruits and seed-pods are used for this purpose and, as recently as 1943, Marie Stopes recommended the use of a plug of wool, soaked in rancid butter, as a wartime expedient. The most sophisticated historical prototype for the modern cervical cap is the eighteenth-century reference[1] to the use of a half lemon, squeezed of its contents, and inserted over the cervix; the residual citric acid, mildly spermicidal, would undoubtedly have provided additional protection.

The earliest commercial and surgical caps had to await the use of crepe, and later vulcanized, rubber and the first medical reference occurs in the German literature where, in 1823, Dr F. A. Wilde describes[2] the use of a cautschuk-pessarium as a 'comfortable and effective' method of birth control. But although an identical article was described and illustrated in the *Lancet* in 1867[3] as a form of treatment for 'anteflexion and anteversion of the uterus' the occlusive cap was not referred to again in the English birth control literature until Allbutt published details in 1887 (see chapter 1, p. 4). By this time the name of Mensinga,[4] a Flensburg physician, had become associated with the device largely through publicity given to it by the Dutch Neo-Malthusians. The development of vulcanized rubber had enabled Mensinga to produce a thinner and more pliable device, within the rim of which was incorporated a flat watchspring and which lay diagonally across the vaginal canal thus occluding both the cervix and the upper part of the vagina.

In England the early birth control clinics followed the Dutch example in adopting the cap as a basic technique. It was not merely appropriate to the female clientele which they aimed at attracting but, in a situation which demanded a maximum of safety, it could be combined with the use of a spermicidal cream to provide a dual method of protection. The two branches of the clinic movement, however, adopted different and 'rival' varieties of the technique which provided the basis for a long and acrimonious disagreement, not merely on the relative efficacy of the methods but also on the question of physiological safety. Marie Stopes' clinic advocated a high-domed cervical cap in combination with greasy suppositories. The clinics of the Society for the Provision of Birth Control Clinics (later the FPA) favoured the spring-rim vaginal diaphragm together with a spermicidal jelly and subsequent douching. Marie Stopes alleged that the diaphragm caused distension of the vaginal muscles whilst the SPBCC replied that the cervical cap produced erosion of the cervix.

Nevertheless, the diaphragm and cap continued to form the basic procedures recommended by the voluntary birth control clinics until the oral contraceptive became available in Britain. Thus, in a survey of all patients attending 315 FPA clinics during November 1960 it was shown that over 95 per cent were offered this form of contraception.[5] It is not, however, a completely acceptable method for all those attending clinics and there is evidence that for many clinic patients the cap is a method of last resort. In the same enquiry it was shown that about four couples try the cap for every three who eventually settle for it.

EXTENT OF CONTEMPORARY USAGE

The diaphragm is like the steam locomotive: it was the first in the field, it brought emancipation to millions, for a long time it had no rivals, it had and still has a large number of devoted supporters; but of late its use has been diminishing and undoubtedly will continue to do so.

At the peak of its popularity the cap and cream method of family planning was used by approximately one in three American couples who tried to plan their families,[6] but in England its use has always been more restricted. In the Population Investigation Committee survey of the use of contraceptives in 1959 it was the method of choice of one in eight of those couples using any method of birth control.[7] It is a method which has always been more likely to be used by school teachers than by shop assistants. Perhaps this is partly an expression of female emancipation and independence and it may arise too from the fact that a diaphragm requires professional medical advice to be correctly fitted.

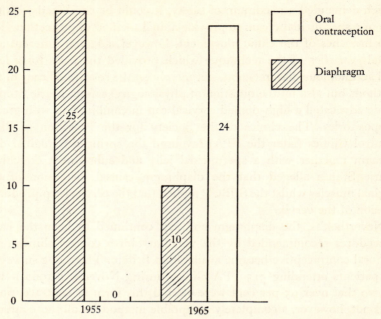

Fig. 6. Usage of diaphragm and oral contraception by white American women.

Many women who have, or might have, used a diaphragm are now using oral contraceptives (figure 6). Although this trend may be expected to continue the method will remain a useful one in the armamentarium of contraceptive procedures.

The failure rate of the cap is closely related to the degree of motivation shown by the woman using it. This is best demonstrated by the increasing effectiveness with which it is used inside marriage as a couple approach, or exceed, what they regard as the ideal size of family. Westoff and co-workers in America (1963) have measured the failure rate of the cap between marriage and the first child, the first and second child and after the second child and correlated this with the number of children the mother said she wanted.[8, 9]

TYPES OF DIAPHRAGM AND RELATED DEVICES

Occlusive caps (figure 7) are not intended as sperm-proof mechanical barriers but are used as vehicles to retain an effective chemical spermicide in contact with the external cervical os. They should always be fitted by a doctor or a specially trained nurse, the woman must be instructed how to use the device and her ability to use it checked. Several types of diaphragm and cap are sold in chemists, surgical goods shops and through mail order firms. The instructions provided are sometimes inaccurate and are too complicated to be followed effectively.

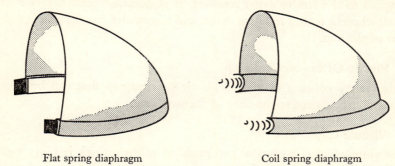

Flat spring diaphragm   Coil spring diaphragm

Fig. 7. Types of diaphragm.

Caps and diaphragms are usually manufactured from rubber and therefore have a finite storage and usage life. They should be stamped with a date of manufacture. They are manufactured under a variety of mysterious and exotic trade names (Appendix III).

1   The Diaphragm (Dutch Cap)

The diaphragm is by far the commonest form of occlusive cap and for most women it is the easiest to fit and use. It is made of fine latex in the form of a thin dome mounted on a thick rim containing a metal spring. The flat spring type is more rigid than the coil spring variety and provides a less easily distorted, more easily inserted device. Diaphragms are manufactured in a series of sizes from 45 mm diameter, rising in steps of 2·5 or 5 mm to 105 mm diameter. The height of the dome varies from maker to maker.

2   Vault Cap

This is a hemispherical rubber or plastic cap which fits in the vaginal vault and closely follows the contours of the cervix. The centre is thin and the rim is thick as with the diaphragm but unlike the diaphragm there is no metal spring in the rim. Vault caps are made in five sizes from 50 to 74 mm.

3 Cervical Caps (Check Pessaries)

These are thimble-shaped rubber caps with thick bases and are de-signed to fit snugly over the cervix. They are manufactured in three or four sizes between 22 and 31 mm. Some cervical caps have a thread attached to the rim to assist removal. It is questionable whether such an attachment makes removal easier and it may deform the inside con-tour of the cap.

4 Plastic Ortho-cervical Cap

This variety consists of a rigid plastic cervical cap that can be worn continuously except at the time of menstruation.

5 Vimule Cap

The vimule cap is a cervical cap made of rubber which is fairly rigid and has a flanged base to increase the degree of suction when the cap is put in place. It is made in 42 and 55 mm sizes.

METHODS OF FITTING

Use of the cap requires at least two appointments, on the first of which it is useful to be able to lend the patient a practice cap. The woman who is going to learn to use a diaphragm or cap must have two qualities, and they are not necessarily related. She must have the intelligence to understand and carry out the correct insertion of the cap and she must have the self-discipline to use it on every occasion she has intercourse. She must not find exploration of her own anatomy distasteful. A woman who has had children is usually more ready to accept the cap than her nulliparous sister. For the woman who is rich, who does not wish to fit her own cap, who cannot or will not accept another method and where both the patient and the doctor have considerable free time it is possible for the practitioner to fit and remove a plastic Ortho-cervical cap with each menstrual cycle.

Having selected the occlusive cap as the most suitable method of family planning the patient is examined, either lying on her back or in the left lateral position. A speculum is passed as part of the normal pelvic examination, and when necessary a smear is taken. The length and position of the cervix is determined, the tone of the perineal muscles and the vaginal wall are examined. The choice of the diaphragm or cap is determined mainly by the findings on pelvic examination. The criteria for using a diaphragm are that:

1. There is no major degree of uterine prolapse.
2. There is good vaginal tone, no marked cystocoele and a defined depression or 'shelf' in the lower part of the vaginal wall behind the symphasis pubis.
3. The patient should be able to feel her own cervix.

The cervical cap and vimule can only be used if:

1. The cervix is readily accessible to the patient.
2. The cervix points forward making it impossible to dislodge the cap during intercourse.
3. The cervix is long enough to hold the cap.
4. The cervix is uneroded and unlacerated.

The vault cap may be the first choice for a patient but more often is used where a diaphragm or cervical cap proves difficult. It is useful in the woman who has some degree of prolapse or poor vaginal tone making a diaphragm difficult to fit, or if the cervix is too short or torn for a cervical cap. In fact, the vault cap is contraindicated if the cervix is too long as it will hold the rim of the cap away from the vaginal vault, making it impossible to establish the necessary degree of suction.

In those rare cases where a woman has an allergy to rubber a plastic vault or cervical cap must be used.

1 Diaphragm

The length of the vagina from the posterior aspect of the symphasis pubis to the posterior fornix is assessed. An appropriate size of diaphragm is selected, the rim is compressed between the thumb and forefinger of the right hand and the diaphragm inserted into the vagina passing the tip along the posterior vaginal wall so that the rim comes to lie in the posterior fornix. The proximal edge of the rim is then pushed up behind the symphasis pubis. The flat spring type of diaphragm is more easily inserted than the coil spring and is more readily placed in the posterior fornix. It is usual to insert the diaphragm dome uppermost.

If correctly positioned the cervix can be felt through the dome of the diaphragm and one finger can just be inserted between the rim of the diaphragm and the symphasis pubis. The woman should not now be aware of the presence of the diaphragm. It is often helpful for the doctor deliberately to place the diaphragm in the wrong position so that the entire device is anterior to the cervix: the patient will then notice some discomfort and find that she can easily feel the rim with her fingers.

To remove the cap the rim is hooked down from behind the symphasis pubis using one finger.

The woman can be taught to insert the diaphragm in one of three positions; lying on her back with her knees drawn up, standing with one foot raised on a chair or toilet seat, or squatting. It is worth enquiring whether the woman uses vaginal tampons as inserting the cap is very similar. Most women find a standing position with one leg raised simplest. The woman is shown how to compress the diaphragm over the first finger by pressure with the middle finger and thumb. Holding the labia apart with her left hand the cap is inserted along the posterior wall of the vagina as far as it will go and keeping it below and behind the cervix (figure 8(a)). The anterior rim of the cap is then tucked up behind the symphasis pubis (figure 8(b)). In the standing position the cap is inserted almost horizontally and in the lying position almost vertically. It is important to make sure that the patient understands the anatomical axis of the vagina is upwards and *backwards*. The lay concept of the vagina is often of a passage placed vertically in the trunk like the lift-shaft in a skyscraper. Unless this idea is corrected the patient will find it difficult to insert the diaphragm and is in danger of placing it anterior to the cervix.

The woman must learn to check that the device is in the correct position. If she has learnt to locate her cervix previously she will be able to feel it through the rubber of the dome of the diaphragm (figure 8(c)). To the woman who is not familiar with her own cervix, it can usefully be described as feeling 'like the tip of your nose'. If the cervix is too remote to feel easily, or the woman has short fingers, or a strong dislike of feeling inside her own vagina and, if there are still reasons why the method is thought suitable, it may be sufficient for the patient to make sure that the anterior rim of the cap is comfortably placed behind the symphasis pubis instead of trying to feel for the cervix.

Some manufacturers supply a diaphragm introducer. This is a plastic rod with a groove at one end and a notch part of the way along its length. The diaphragm is compressed, fitted into the grooved end and hooked over the notch. The introducer is passed along the posterior wall of the vagina below and beyond the cervix as before. The introducer is disengaged by giving it a quarter turn to the right or left. The anterior

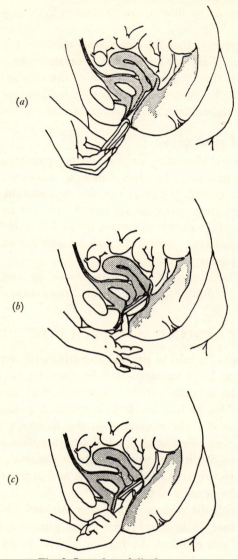

(a)

(b)

(c)

Fig. 8. Insertion of diaphragm.

rim of the diaphragm still has to be pushed up behind the pubic bone and the position checked by feeling the cervix through the rubber dome. Like the invention of the knife and fork, it can make the procedure which is being undertaken easier and more attractive but it is difficult to improve on the human hand.

The patient should be shown how to remove the cap with her hooked finger.

It must be explained that the cap is only effective when used with a spermicidal cream. Three or four inches of cream (a teaspoonful) should be squeezed from the tube onto the side of the diaphragm which will be against the cervix. Some of the cream should be spread round the rim and this has the additional advantage of making insertion easier.

2   Cervical and vault caps

Caps are more rigid than diaphragms and are partly held in place by suction. The patient must be shown how to manoeuvre the cap into position over the cervix. When in use the caps should be about one-third filled with contraceptive cream but the patient must be told not to use too much cream as this will make it difficult to obtain the correct degree of suction. Extra spermicide may be added from an applicator or inserted as a pessary.

The cap can be removed by the fingers or by a thread if one is attached. When properly fitted it should be quite difficult to remove.

TEACHING AND FOLLOW UP

The patient should be told to practise inserting and removing the diaphragm or cap, to leave the appliance in place for several hours at a time and to make sure that it does not move out of position if she empties her bladder or has her bowels open. A practice cap or diaphragm can be used without cream but the woman must understand that it will not be an effective method of contraception until the device and her ability to use it correctly have been checked. She should be asked to make a return visit in about a week and to put the cap in place before keeping the appointment.

At the check visit the woman should be examined with the appliance in place. In the case of the diaphragm it is not unusual to find that the wrong size has been fitted at the first visit. The woman, especially if nulliparous, may have been slightly tense at the first visit, and a larger size of diaphragm may now be needed. The doctor or nurse should check that the diaphragm covers the cervix and make sure that the woman has been checking the device correctly. The patient should be asked if the diaphragm is comfortable or whether she is aware of it at any time. She can be told that her husband is most unlikely to feel the diaphragm. Vault and cervical caps are checked in a similar way, although, since they do not depend upon vaginal muscular tone for correct fitting the size will not need changing unless the fit was mis-judged at the first visit. It may be wise to warn the woman that the vault cap can sometimes be felt by the husband during intercourse but that it should not cause any real annoyance.

USE AND CARE

Careful teaching about the use and care of a cap or diaphragm is as important as correct fitting. The patient must be reminded about the way in which the cap holds a spermicidal cream in relation to the neck of the womb and told that sperm remain capable of fertilizing the egg for many hours after they have been placed in the vagina. The necessity to use it at every intercourse needs re-emphasizing and the doctor as well as the patient must be prepared to make some assessment of how well the method is likely to be used in the long run. Some patients may prefer to put the device in every night as a routine, like brushing the teeth.

The cap can be put in place up to two hours before having inter-course. If it is put in close to the time of coitus it is important that it should be inserted before any sexual play takes place. The appliance must remain in place for a minimum of six hours after intercourse and it can remain in place much longer. In practice it is usually inserted on going to bed and taken out next morning. If the cap is inserted several hours before intercourse or if a second intercourse takes place soon after the first, spermicidal cream should be added with an applicator or in-serted in pessary form. A pessary takes some time to melt at body temperature and should be inserted about 15 min before coitus.

A suitable spermicidal cream should be provided. The choice is a wide one (Appendix III). Some creams will discolour rubber but pro-vided the cap is cleansed after use any of the spermicides on the IPPF and FPA lists can be used and the choice is usually made according to whether or not the woman says that she needs a cream which will also act as a lubricant. A woman may try several varieties of cream before finding one that she likes best. Women will find that creams are cheaper when bought from clinics or doctors. If the cap is used in domiciliary family planning practice the spermicide must usually be provided free or a desire to economise may lead to failure of the method.

After use the cap should be washed in warm water. Excess heat should be avoided, if soap is used it should be a mild, unscented variety and all antiseptic solutions must be forbidden. The cap should be dried, dusted with talcum powder and replaced in its container. The patient should learn to examine her own cap: at intervals it should be held up in front of a good light or filled with water to see if there are thin patches or holes. Flaws are most likely to develop near the rim of a diaphragm and if the rubber in this region becomes puckered the diaphragm needs changing. The dome should not be stretched and the woman who is not a full-time housewife should take care about long finger nails piercing the rubber during handling. Plastic caps are more robust than rubber ones but may crack with age.

A patient with a diaphragm or cap should be seen by a doctor or trained nurse once a year and should have the opportunity of returning more often if she wishes. A newly married girl, or a girl beginning regular premarital intercourse, should be seen after about three months. Domiciliary patients may need checking much more often. Women should also be seen after a pregnancy, after any pelvic operation or if they have experienced a substantial change in weight (10 lb or more).

At all times the doctor should be ready to answer questions and give explanations. The woman may need reassurance that the appliance cannot get lost inside her, or that it will not cause infection. Some women believe the vagina is a germ-free place and it may be useful to point out the other unsterile things that are normally placed in it. A woman may need to be told that if menstruation occurs with a cap in place it will not do her any harm. If the woman is in the habit of douching she should be told not to do this until the cap has been removed.

EVALUATION

The diaphragm, like the condom, is an entirely harmless method of birth control and has no medical side effects. Compared with the condom it has the advantage of being fitted and removed remote from intercourse, but it is more complicated to use. It leaves the control of pregnancy entirely in the hands of the woman and it is reasonably safe when carefully used.

Inside many marriages it is a very suitable method of spacing a family. In fact, it can be deliberately misused to solve the problem of the woman who emotionally wants another child but cannot say so rationally. It is possible, and in some cases easy, to fit a virgin with a diaphragm. But there is no evidence to suggest that the use of a diaphragm, compared with other methods of contraception, either helps or hinders sexual adjustment in early marriage. From the reverse point of view, one should perhaps be cautious in fitting a cap in a girl who may have sexual problems.

The cap can be the contraceptive method of choice for some women when they have completed their family but it must be recognized that many women find the cap distasteful and others abandon its regular use because they find it messy or tiresome. It is a middle-class method of contraception, being used by the wives of professional, managerial and white-collar workers. Except among a minority who are highly motivated, it has never been widely used by the wives of manual workers or unskilled labourers. Non-acceptance of the method goes with a complex of sexual taboos, which are still widespread in British society, such as reluctance for a wife to be seen nude by her husband, a sense of shame at breast feeding before others and a strong desire to check genital play in infants. To extend the last example, nine out of ten wives of unskilled labourers are disturbed if their children 'play with themselves' and will smack the child or try to stop the habit in some other way, whereas only a quarter of the wives of professional men bother to try to prevent such activities.[10] It is not difficult to see that this type of attitude may be associated with a refusal on the part of the mother to use a cap, or she may use it badly and inconsistently.

To proselytize the use of the cap can be dangerous. An anatomically perfect fit is of no value if the woman has not the inclination or opportunity to use it every time she has intercourse. Even a mild degree of aversion is bad. In a study of criminal abortions in Amsterdam, Treffers[11] found that among women who had become pregnant and subsequently had a criminal abortion the failure rate with the diaphragm had been 60 per HWY. In a control group of women who had become pregnant but had not resorted to abortion the failure rate was 20 per HWY.

7 CHEMICAL CONTRACEPTIVES

HISTORY AND CONTEMPORARY USAGE

Most contemporary vaginal contraceptives rely for their effectiveness on both chemical and physical properties. The spermicidal component, whose purpose is to immobilize the spermatozoa, is invariably combined with a gelatinous or oleaginous base which tends to form a barrier to penetration and provides a vehicle to carry the spermicide. Traditional pessaries produced from gums, resins and vegetable substances had this predominantly physical mode of action; any spermicidal power which they possessed was adventitious. Scientific interest in birth control during the late nineteenth century was quickly directed to increasing the specifically chemical activity of vaginal products and this property became even more important with the increasing use of an additional barrier in the form of a cap or diaphragm.

It is perhaps predictable that quinine, in view of its ubiquitous role in the *materia medica* of the period, should have been the earliest compound to be used as a spermicide. The credit for its adaptation to this use belongs to a Clerkenwell pharmacist, W. J. Rendell, whose name has been associated with vaginal contraception in England for four generations. In 1885 Rendell evolved[1] a soluble cocoa-butter suppository containing quinine sulphate which he marketed in red slide boxes bearing a facsimile of his signature. These suppositories achieved a considerable popularity and before the end of the century they were sold by virtually every pharmacy in the country. These suppositories have continued to be sold to the present day—still in the same red box. Nor was any change made in the original formula until 1960 except for a period during the Second World War when, due to government restrictions on the supply of quinine, hexyl resorcinol was substituted as the spermicidal ingredient.

This change was quickly followed by large numbers of complaints of failure which did much to sustain the myth that every packet contained an ineffective item. A sociologist carrying out a survey of working-class

74

families during this period noted[2] how frequently the expression 'This is a [Rendell's] baby' cropped up in interview. The volume of sales for this product declined by 30 per cent and recovered only when quinine again became available at the end of the war. In 1960 an entirely new formula was introduced but the wartime experiences were undoubtedly responsible for a decline in the popularity of this method of contraception.

The family planning movement had an interest in chemical contraception as a part of its combined cap/cream or diaphragm/jelly regime. Just as the early movement in England was divided on the subject of vaginal or cervical caps there were differences, too, on the relative merits of different chemical products, the Marie Stopes' clinics favouring chinosol with a cocoa-butter formulation and the SPBCC recommending quinine with gelatine base.[3] One of the first tasks of the early research committee of the family planning movement was to initiate an investigation into chemical spermicides and the result of this was Volpar, a series of products including paste and gels containing phenyl mercuric acetate as the spermicidal ingredient. Although an advance on the existing formulations, and still one of the most effective products currently available, Volpar is by no means the perfect chemical spermicide and it is likely that a modest outlay on research in this field could result in the elaboration of more effective compounds.

The only other purpose-developed spermicidal compound is p-triisopropylphenoxypolyethoxyethanol which is widely used in the United States in a number of proprietary formulations. There and elsewhere, however, the majority of commercial preparations are based on quinine, boric acid, lactic acid, chinosol, hexyl resorcinol, ricinoleic acid and formaldehyde. All of these are used in the four major classes of vaginal compound: suppositories, jellies, creams and foams.

TYPES AVAILABLE

1 Chemical Suppositories

Suppositories, pessaries, gels or 'solubles' as they are variously known are the most convenient, and least reliable, of all forms of chemical contraception. Consisting of 4 to 5 g of a soap, gelatine or cocoa-butter base with a chemical spermicide incorporated, they are designed for insertion shortly before intercourse and are, if they are to be effective, required to melt quickly at body temperature. Even where reliance can

75

be placed on adequate melting it is unlikely that a single suppository will achieve the degree of dispersion within the vagina which is possible with creams and jellies.

The main advantages of suppositories are their ready availability and ease of use. A survey[4] in Britain in 1966 revealed that there were more than fifty brands on sale in either surgical stores and chemists or by mail order. In a number of cases the instructions omitted to state for how long they remained effective and this form of chemical contraception was associated with a number of wild and extravagant claims, e.g. 'treble strength' and 'recommended by the elite of the medical profession'. In general, suppositories represent inferior value, weight for weight, in comparison with the equivalent cream or jelly product.

2 Contraceptive Jellies

In the contraceptive jelly the spermicidal ingredient is made up in a gelatinous base which is water-soluble and easily dispersed within the vagina and which liquefies at a lower temperature than most creams. For this reason it is more suitable for the woman with inadequate secretions. Mercuric compounds are more generally made up in a jelly base: with other compounds there is usually no difference, either in the spermicidal capacity or in the speed with which the spermicide is liberated, between jelly and cream.

3 Creams or Pastes

With these products the base consists of a stearate soap which is alleged to adhere more easily to membranous tissues and thus provide a more persisting barrier. There is, however, little difference in either reliability or cost between creams and jellies; most manufacturers produce both cream and jelly equivalents and the latter appears to be slightly more popular for every brand.

4 Foams and Aerosols

The theoretical advantages of foam over other chemical contraceptives lie in the fact that, in addition to the action of the spermicidal agent, the effervescent mass produced when the ingredients come into contact with moisture consitutes a more dense physical barrier occluding the os uterus. It has also been claimed that the process of effervescence forces the active agent into those interstices where live spermatozoa might otherwise remain.

Foam contraceptives were first developed in Germany in the early 1920s and from 1927 were marketed in England by Coates and Cooper under the trade name Speton. A small, but apparently persisting, minority of couples has continued to use foam contraceptives. In the PIC survey it was found[5] that 1·9 per cent of women married in the 1930s, 3·1 per cent of those married in the 1940s and 3·7 per cent of those married in the 1950s used this form of contraception. Amongst the couples married in 1965 who were interviewed in the Hull Marriage Survey less than 1 per cent mentioned foam as their major method of contraception. According[6] to the most recent *Which?* report Gynomin, manufactured by Coates and Cooper, is the most readily available of the nine brands on the English market. Foam is apparently even less popular in the United States than in England despite the greater use there of female methods generally.

Like the IUD, foam appears to have passed into relative obscurity during the pre-war and immediate post-war period until the Population Council, in its search for a simple method of contraception for use in underdeveloped countries, revived an interest in it during the 1950s.[7] In an early clinical trial in the United States foam tablets were given to 250 couples of low socio-economic status with control groups using jelly and diaphragms. The results were hardly encouraging.[8] The pregnancy rate was 22·5 per HWY and a large number of couples complained about burning sensation and messiness.

Nevertheless many subsequent trials have been undertaken. In England the Council for the Investigation of Fertility Control (CIFC) financed a series of tests by Mears which were even less satisfactory than the Population Council trials. Of 670 volunteers only 400 completed the trial and amongst these a pregnancy rate of 37 per HWY was reported.[9]

In spite of these relatively disastrous results the Population Council, the IPPF and other organizations have persisted in their attempt to popularize the foam tablet, apparently on the grounds that, notwithstanding its high failure rate, it is a readily acceptable, safe and simple method of contraception suited particularly to use in countries where these factors may be more important than maximum reliability. Thus, in a paper given at the World Population Conference in Belgrade in 1965, a participant explained:[10] 'This method is mainly favoured [in the Arab Republic] by illiterate women, especially in rural areas, for simplicity of usage. It has a high demand from users of birth control in spite of its lower rate of success than the diaphragm and jelly.' Foam was given a major mention in at least eleven papers presented in Belgrade —always in connection with its use in underdeveloped areas.

The introduction of aerosols gave a fresh, but apparently temporary, impetus to the interest in foam contraception. The incorporation of a butane propellant into an effective spermicidal cream would appear to offer considerable advantages and one such product, Emko, became available in England during the course of the CIFC trial, the later stages of which were used to evaluate the product against two foam tablets. Emko was found to be a more efficient, but not a more acceptable, product than either of the others but the pregnancy rate was still higher than that of traditional methods. In reporting these results Mears promised[11] a new trial in which Emko would be compared with the condom and the diaphragm, but this was never undertaken by CIFC largely because the relative expensiveness of the product did not appear to justify its marginal superiority over foam tablets.

In recent years the interest in foam appears to have waned, even in relation to its overseas use, owing to the attention now being given to the IUD. Occasional journal articles still appear reporting new trials and in a number of countries foam tablets have been included as an available choice in 'cafeteria' programmes of contraceptive provision; Egypt has recently set up a factory for the manufacture of foam tablets. In advanced countries it may, because of its high acceptability, continue to play a very minor part in the general pattern of contraceptive usage.

USE AND APPLICATION

Suppositories are the easiest form of contraceptive method and require no instruction apart from the warning that multiple or prolonged coitus requires plural insertion. When contraceptive creams and jellies are used in conjunction with a diaphragm or cap they should be liberally applied to the device before insertion. When used as a supplement to the condom or alone, jellies, pastes and foams are usually and most conveniently applied by means of a plunger type applicator into which the paste is squeezed, or the foam impelled, the syringe being subsequently voided as far into the vagina as possible. It is important that the material should be deposited anterior to the cervix and, in the case of a woman whose posterior fornix is unusually deep, this may require some additional care.

Otherwise, the only instructions necessary relate to elementary hygiene and cleanliness and the need for additional insertions when repeated intercourse takes place.

EVALUATION

The main advantages of chemical contraceptives are their ready availability and ease of application. Strictly, they should always be used in conjunction with cap, diaphragm or condom but, used alone, they are better than nothing. The high acceptability of chemical products outweighs their relatively high failure rate and in some underdeveloped countries they are likely, therefore, to provide a continuing focus of interest for family planning programmes. Their effectiveness could undoubtedly be improved by basic research on spermicidal compounds.

8 THE SAFE PERIOD

HISTORY AND EXTENT OF USE

Attempts to avoid conception by the practice of timed periodic abstinence have been undertaken in most societies of which we have historical or anthropological knowledge. The most common of these involve the avoidance of intercourse before, during or after menstruation and from ancient Rome, through the Indian cultures of New Mexico to the Nandi of East Africa, variations on this practice have been reported.[1] Nineteenth-century Europe was no exception and in 1853 tacit Vatican approval[2] coincided with the development of a spurious scientific analogy resulting in a popularization of the idea that the menstrual phase represented the period of peak fecundity and that an infertile period occurred in the middle of the cycle.

The Bishop of Amiens had asked the Sacred Penitentiary how he should deal with those couples amongst his flock who were confining intercourse to the *tempus ageneseos* and was advised not to interfere 'so long as they do nothing to impede conception'. In the same year Theodor Bischoff succeeded in recovering eggs from the tubes and uteri of bitches during heat and was led to assume an identity between oestrous vaginal bleeding in domestic mammals and menstruation in women. The theological morality of confining intercourse to this cruelly mistaken interval of assumed infertility was reaffirmed in a Vatican statement of 1880 and late nineteenth- and early twentieth-century birth control literature continued to publicize this erroneous interpretation of the 'safe period'. Thus Allbutt, in *The Wife's Handbook*, advised abstention from intercourse from 5 days before to 8 days after menstruation and this was repeated by almost every subsequent writer until the 1930s.

Since the phase of the cycle to which intercourse was being confined was precisely the period of maximum fecundity (and which is today recommended as such to the subfertile) it is hardly surprising that the method achieved neither success nor popularity. Of the first 234 patients attending the Liverpool family planning clinic in 1927 not one mentioned the safe period as a previously used technique.

Accumulating knowledge on human ovulation, resulting from observations made at laparotomy, from primate studies and from increased information on menstrual physiology, provided the basis for a re-evaluation during the 1930s of the concept of the infertile period. In 1929 Knaus, in Austria and Ogino, in Japan, independently proposed[3],[4] a regime based on the assumption that ovulation would occur 14 days before the onset of the next menstruation and the consequent avoidance of intercourse during the mid-cycle phase. The validity of their hypothesis was subsequently confirmed by the recovery of eggs and early ova from women with known menstrual and coital histories.[5]

The Ogino–Knaus theory, as it quickly became known, was enthusiastically taken up by Roman Catholic doctors during the 1930s and a flood of books appeared expounding the 'non-contraceptive method of birth regulation' and 'lawful birth control according to nature's laws'. By 1955 one-fifth of all American couples practising birth control had used this method[6] and in the 1959 PIC survey in England 16 per cent of informants were found to have practised it at some time.[7] The recent popularity of the IUD and the oral contraceptive have resulted in a decline in the number of couples using the rhythm method and in the most recent surveys the percentage in the US had dropped to 13[8] and in England to 7.[9]

THE RHYTHM PROCEDURE

The 'safe period' or rhythm method of birth control restricts intercourse to the period of physiological sterility in each menstrual cycle. It is based on the premise that, in general circumstances, the ovary expels only one ovum per cycle and that this is available for fertilization for only 24 hours. Spermatozoa, once they have entered the uterus, can remain viable for only 48 hours and there is thus a minimum period of only 3 days in each cycle during which conception is theoretically possible. If intercourse is omitted during this time pregnancy will be avoided.

In practice the fertile period is considerably lengthened both by the fact that few women menstruate with complete regularity and by the degree of uncertainty which attaches to the precise day of ovulation in even the most predictable series of cycles. For although Ogino and

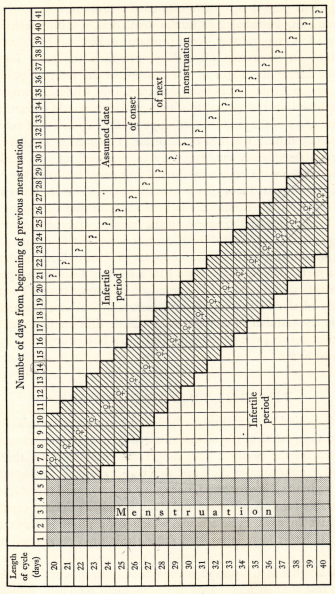

Fig. 9. Ovulation chart for cycles of 20 to 40 days in length.

Knaus had assumed that ovulation would ideally occur on the 14th day before the next menstruation they recognized that this was subject to a variation of two days in either direction. For practical purposes, therefore, days 12 to 16 (always counting backwards from the expected date of the next menstruation) are regarded as possible ovulatory days and the basis of the fertile period. To these are then added days 17 and 18, for previously deposited spermatozoa, and day 11, which represents the limit of ovum survival. (The Catholic Marriage Advisory Council recommends the further inclusion of days 10 and 19 but the marginal gain in safety is hardly proportional to the inconvenience which this would involve.)

These 8 days which constitute the fertile period and which are illustrated for cycles of 20 to 40 days in length in figure 9 bear a constant relationship to the onset of the next menstruation but the precise date of this event can never, of course, be accurately predicted. For birth control purposes, however, it is the determination of the limits of the two phases of the infertile period which is most important and for this it is sufficient to know only the earliest possible and latest possible dates on which the next period could occur. These are obtained by calculating back from data obtained from the study of the past menstrual history of the individual woman who, before she begins to use the rhythm method, must keep records for at least six months and, if possible, for a year. Counting the first day of bleeding in each cycle as day 1 she is then able to furnish information which will reveal the likely length of her longest and shortest cycles.

To calculate the pre-ovulatory days which may be expected to be infertile 18 is subtracted from the shortest recorded cycle; similarly, the infertile days in the luteal phase are determined by subtracting 11 from the longest cycle. Thus, in the case of a woman whose cycles ranged from 25 to 32 days, the 'safe period' would extend up to day 7 (i.e. $25-18=7$) and from day 21 (i.e. $32-11=21$) onwards. Figure 10 shows the standard chart from which such calculations can quickly be made by women possessing only the minimum degree of numeracy. Intending users of the rhythm method should be instructed to mark a calendar, once the relevant calculations have been made, on the first day of every period, crossing through the fertile days. The marked calendar should, of course, be shown to the husband.

The calendar technique depends for its effectiveness on a rough prediction of a future, and therefore uncertain, event: it is rather like

Length of shortest period	First 'unsafe' day after start of any period	Length of longest period	Last 'unsafe' day after start of any period
20 days	2nd day	20 days	9th day
21 days	3rd day	21 days	10th day
22 days	4th day	22 days	11th day
23 days	5th day	23 days	12th day
24 days	6th day	24 days	13th day
25 days	7th day	25 days	14th day
26 days	8th day	26 days	15th day
27 days	9th day	27 days	16th day
28 days	10th day	28 days	17th day
29 days	11th day	29 days	18th day
30 days	12th day	30 days	19th day
31 days	13th day	31 days	20th day
32 days	14th day	32 days	21st day
33 days	15th day	33 days	22nd day
34 days	16th day	34 days	23rd day
35 days	17th day	35 days	24th day
36 days	18th day	36 days	25th day
37 days	19th day	37 days	26th day
38 days	20th day	38 days	27th day
39 days	21st day	39 days	28th day
40 days	22nd day	40 days	29th day

Fig. 10. The rhythm method—how to calculate the 'safe' and 'unsafe' days.

selecting university students on the basis of A-level examinations which they have not yet taken. It is quite unsuitable for women with cycles of less than 20 days in length or whose cycles vary by more than 10 days. An alternative to the calendar technique which aims to pinpoint more effectively the actual day of ovulation is the temperature method. This is based on the fact that progesterone produces a rise in the basic metabolic rate and a corresponding rise in body temperature, usually of the order of 0·6 °F. Consequently, ovulation may be determined retrospectively by daily temperature recordings. But it must be noted that the changes are slight, easy to misinterpret without considerable teaching and liable to be confused by intercurrent illness. Moreover, many women either find it difficult to read a clinical thermometer or are incapable of shaking the mercury down.

For those women who appear anxious to use the method careful instruction is necessary. The temperature must be taken on waking and before the woman undertakes any physical activity. She must have been at rest for at least one hour (a contingency which must be rarely possible for a multiparous woman with a young family) and must neither smoke nor drink before taking her temperature. If the temperature is to be taken orally this should be carried out with the lips closed for three minutes and with the thermometer bulb resting under the tongue and in contact with the floor of the mouth. Oral temperatures may not be sufficiently accurate and 'taking the temperature rectally (in the back passage) gives the most reliable curve and one that is easiest...to inter-

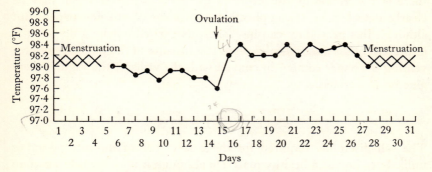

Fig. 11. Temperature curve showing ovulatory rise.

pret. The method is quite simple. Dip the bulb of the thermometer in a jar of vaseline petroleum jelly kept specially for this purpose and gently insert the bulb into the rectum as you are lying in bed. It should be left in position for THREE minutes by the clock and then removed and read immediately.'[10]

The temperature curve shown in figure 11 is an ideal which may vary widely in practice. For this reason it is essential that the first interpretation of temperature curves, based on the records of at least three complete cycles, should be carried out by the doctor. Only when he is satisfied that the woman is capable of taking her own temperature and of understanding the results should she be allowed to rely on the rhythm method alone. In this case she should be instructed to postpone intercourse for three days after the temperature has reached luteal level. If a slow or irregular rise is recorded, intercourse should not take place until five days after the rise began and if the temperature rises, drops and rises again calculations should be made from the start of the second rise. Care should be taken to avoid the muddling effects of intercurrent infection. If an anovulatory cycle occurs the use of the method compels abstinence at the only time when intercourse would have been totally safe.

85

The temperature method is an attempt, if a bothersome one, to pinpoint more accurately than is possible with the calendar the precise date of ovulation. If some physiological or biochemical correlate of the changes immediately preceding ovulation could be discovered the 'safe period' would become a much more satisfactory method of contraception. A biochemical technique which crops up in the literature with almost rhythmic regularity is the cervical enzyme test. During ovulation there is a secretion of glucose from the cervical glands which may be clearly detected by the application of a strip of enzyme paper. But although this procedure can be effectively carried out by a doctor it is impracticable as a self-administered test because of the difficulty of preventing the paper coming in contact with the walls of the vagina where glucose is secreted.

SIDE EFFECTS

The self-discipline required for the correct use of the safe period is unlikely to impair a healthy marriage although it may exclude a certain amount of rightful pleasure. A few couples who have had strong religious motivations have even reported the method to be beneficial in sexual adjustment. On the other hand a poor marriage, especially between people of low intelligence who find it difficult to plan ahead, can be wrecked by the frustrations and failures of the rhythm method.

Two medical complications resulting from the use of the safe period deserve consideration. Some ectopic pregnancies may follow conception late in the menstrual cycle with failure to inhibit the next period and consequent displacement of the ovum to an extrauterine site or an abnormal intrauterine attachment (e.g. placenta previa). This hypothesis is supported by the fact that spontaneous ectopic pregnancies occur only in animals which menstruate and by statistical analyses of embryonic and fetal size in ectopic pregnancies. If it is correct the safe period may predispose to abnormal gestation.[11]

The systematic disjunction of the time of ovulation and the time of coitus and the consequent likelihood that accidental conception will involve either an ageing ovum or a deteriorating sperm significantly increases the chances of embryonic abnormalities. The high incidence of anencephaly and spina bifida in Catholic populations has recently been attributed to the attempted use of the rhythm.[12] The feasibility of this assumption finds support in the low rate of fetal abnormalities amongst orthodox Jews (amongst whom there is complete abstinence from intercourse for seven days after menstruation) and by the successful treatment of cases of repeated abortion, repeated miscarriage and repeated fetal abnormalities by preconceptional profertility regimen in which intercourse is confined to the anticipated date of ovulation.

EVALUATION

The sole advantage of the rhythm method over other forms of contraception is that it is the only method positively approved by the Roman Catholic Church and a number of Catholics may therefore wish to rely on it. Provided the woman avoids buying any complicated calculators (which are totally unnecessary) the method is without financial cost. Tietze, Poliakoff and Rock have suggested that 'The rhythm method offers a satisfactory degree of protection against unwanted pregnancy to rigorously selected and carefully instructed wives who, with their husbands, are intelligent and strongly motivated. For others and for those to whom pregnancy would be dangerous, the effectiveness of the method is not considered adequate.'[13]

The 'satisfactory degree' of protection referred to here is overstated because the authors have, in evaluating the use-effectiveness of the method, overlooked the important fact referred to in chapter 3, that the period of exposure for users of the rhythm method is drastically reduced. Nevertheless, they are correct in pointing out that the reliability of the method is proportional to the intelligence and self-discipline of the couple practising it and if either rhythm or temperature method has been used for many years with success and satisfaction there is little reason to advise a change. If, on the other hand, a woman wants to try the method it is worth considering in those cases where the couple are intelligent, have not already had as many or more children than they want and where the woman has a reasonably regular cycle.

The method is contraindicated in menopausal women with irregular cycles and those for whom an unplanned pregnancy would be disastrous. It is useless during lactation, although conception may occur before the menses are re-established and it is unreliable in the first three or four cycles that recur. Often it fails in the woman who most needs to avoid pregnancy and where there has been one mistake, owing either to the physiological inappropriateness of the woman's cycle or to the psychological unsuitability of the couple, the chances of further unwanted pregnancies are increased.

Although the method, requiring no mechanical aids, should be applicable to all situations in which coitus is possible it appears to be especially likely to fail whilst the couple are on holiday. This is almost certainly because of an increase in coital activity on such occasions and this widely observed, yet seemingly irrelevant, phenomenon illustrates the interplay of two statistical probabilities in 'Vatican roulette': the chance of pregnancy resulting from a single act of intercourse and the chance of ovulation occurring within a predetermined period.

de Bethune[14] has analysed the statistical basis of child spacing and explored the predicted interval between two births according to different probabilities that a non-pregnant and normally fecund woman can go through a single specified monthly cycle without conceiving: a monthly security factor named after Pope Pius XII's 1951 Address 'una base sufficientemente sicura'. If the desired interval between two births is 12 months the monthly security factor must equal 0·8; if the desired interval is two years 0·96 and if 60 months 0·99. Using published data on the effectiveness of the rhythm method, and assuming that the fertile period lasts only 12 hours, a couple who want a two-year spacing interval are limited statistically to two acts of coitus per cycle and a couple seeking a four-year interval to a maximum of one act of coitus per cycle. 'It is not surprising', concludes the author, 'that the rhythm method has become a source of mental torture to many couples.'

9 ORAL CONTRACEPTIVES

HISTORICAL

In 1897 Beard suggested that the corpus luteum inhibited ovulation during pregnancy and by the early years of this century the role of the ovaries in the sexual cycle was partly understood. In 1912 Fellner studied the effect of injections of ovarian extracts and showed they promoted uterine and mammary growth. Oestrogen and progesterone were isolated in the 1930s and in 1936 MacCorquodale, Thayer and Doisy extracted 25 mg of pure crystalline 17β-oestradiol from four tons of sows' ovaries.[1]

The role of the pituitary in controlling the ovarian cycle was elucidated in the 1920s and in 1932 Moore and Price gave an account of the pituitary feedback mechanism. The possibility of inhibiting ovulation then became apparent and in 1933 Hartman suggested to a colleague that 'amniotin' (a preparation of oestrogens from bovine amniotic fluid) might be used as a contraceptive. In 1940 Sturgis and Albright reported that the use of oestrogen by injection relieved painful dysmenorrhea and inhibited ovulation.[2]

Acceptable, effective and readily available oral contraception required a cheap source of steroids that could be given orally. Steroids of plant origin can be obtained in large quantities and in the late 1930s Russell Marker synthesized progesterone in this way. In 1943 he offered his skills to a commercial organization in Mexico, that was to become the Syntex corporation. The impact which the preparation of steroid hormones from plant sources made can be gauged by the fact that Marker is said to have presented as his credentials two jars filled with four and a half pounds of progesterone—worth about $160,000 at the then market price. By 1950 steroid hormones were available at one-hundredth their price a decade previously.

In 1938 ethisterone was found to be weakly active when given by mouth and in 1956 Syntex patented *norethisterone* (known as *norethindrone* in the USA) which proved to be a most potent oral progestational agent. The earliest trials of norethisterone on women were by Rock, Pincus and Garcia[3] and it proved an effective contraceptive, but the endometrium tended to be shed at irregular times in the menstrual cycle and in order to control this 'breakthrough bleeding' an oestrogen was added. The combination of another progestagen, norethynodrel, and of mestranol was marketed as Enavid by the Searle Company in 1957 and came to be widely used in the United States in 1959. It was approved by the Family Planning Association of Great Britain in 1960. Large-scale field trials have been conducted in Puerto Rico since 1956. In 1963 Goldzieher and his co-workers introduced a sequential regime of oestrogen alone for part of the cycle followed by oestrogen and a progestagen.[4]

The Pill has gained a new significance in the language as well as in the lives of women and is widely used to describe combined and serial preparations.

NATURAL AND ARTIFICIAL
OVARIAN HORMONES

The carbon atoms making up a steroid molecule are numbered according to the convention shown below in figure 12. Oestrogens contain 18 carbon atoms, androgens 19 and progesterone 21. The textbook method of illustrating the carbon skeleton of the steroid molecule obscures its true three-dimensional structure. Isomers differing in biological activity can be obtained by substitutions of hydrogen atoms. Side chains projecting above the plane of the ring are designated β and represented by a solid line of the structural formulae, and those below the plane of the ring as α and represented by a dotted line.

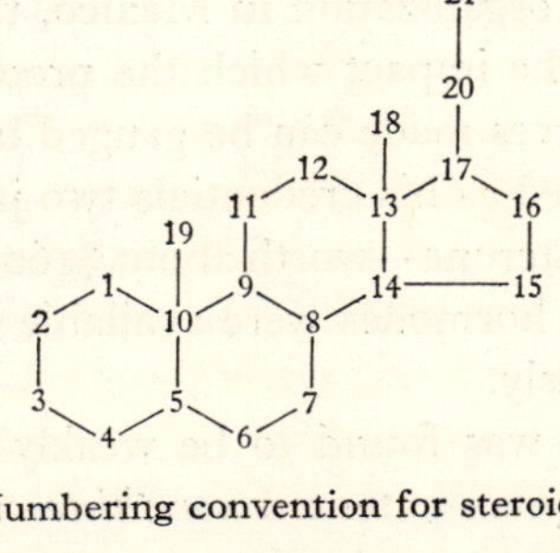

Fig. 12. Numbering convention for steroid molecule.

1   Oestrogens

In the female, oestrogens are produced by the ovaries and placenta and, in the male, by the testicular interstitial cells and from the breakdown of testosterone. In both sexes they are produced by the adrenal cortex. Oestrogens are conjugated as water-soluble sulphates and glucuronides in the liver and excreted in the urine.

During the proliferative phase of the human menstrual cycle 17β-oestradiol (figure 13) and oestrone can be extracted from human ovaries

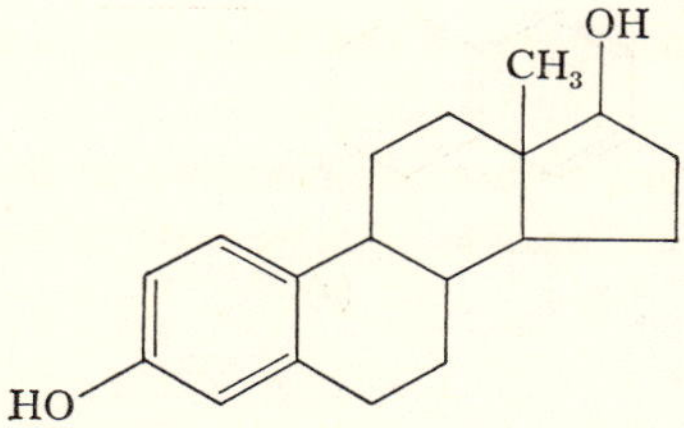

Fig. 13. 17β-oestradiol.

and during the secretory phase oestradiol is also present. 17β-oestradiol and oestrone have been extracted from the ovarian vein blood with difficulty so most knowledge of the normal output of oestrogens is derived from the chromatographic study of urinary oestrogens. About 20 per cent of the total oestrogen secreted appears in the urine as oestriol, oestrone and oestradiol. In the normal ovulatory cycle output is lowest in the first week, rises to a peak at the time of ovulation and is maintained at an elevated level for the remainder of the cycle.

Oestrogens are responsible for endometrial proliferation and, with progesterone, for the secretory phase. In some animals they are necessary for ovo-implantation. Oestrogens inhibit follicle-stimulating hormone (FSH) secretion but stimulate the release of luteinizing hormone (LH). These effects are mediated by the hypothalamus and the pituitary portal system. If the pituitary is transplanted to a different site cyclical ovarian function ceases, but returns if the transplant is replaced under the median eminence of the hypothalamus and revascularized. Oestrogens cause sodium, chloride and water retention but, unlike androgens, have little effect on nitrogen metabolism. The concentration of cholesterol in the α-lipoprotein fraction of plasma is increased and that in the β-lipoprotein fraction reduced. They have little effect on the growth of epiphysial cartilage but promote fusion. In the breasts they cause secretion in the ducts and oedema of the stromal tissue.

A variety of oral and injectable preparations of oestrogen is available but only two are used in oral contraceptives. Both have an ethinyl ($-C\equiv CH$) group in the α-position at carbon 17 which is thought to be responsible for their effectiveness when taken orally (figure 14).

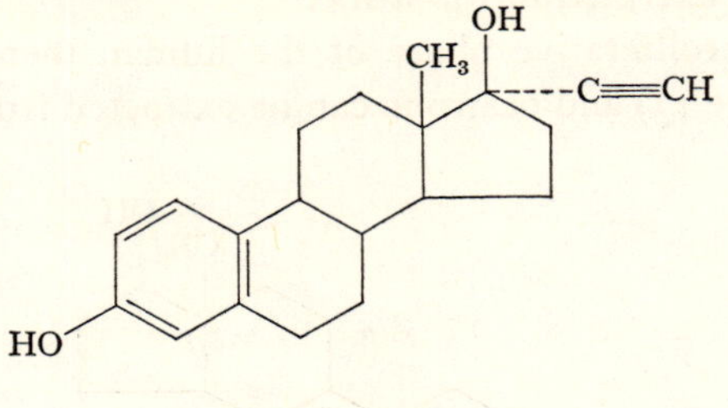

(a)

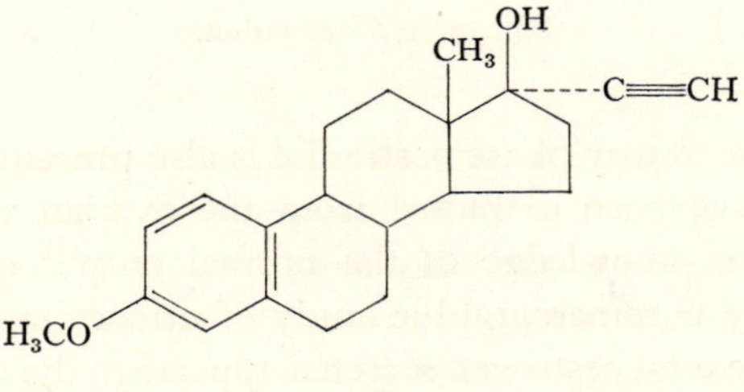

(b)

Fig. 14. Oestrogens used in oral contraceptives. (a) Ethynyloestradiol: Combination tablets—Anovlar; Anovlar-21; Gynovlar; Volidan; Provest; Norlestrin. Sequential tablets—Serial-28. (b) Mestranol: Combination tablets—Conovid; Conovid-E; Lyndiol; Lyndiol-2·5; Orthonovin; Ovulen-1 mg; Previson. Sequential tablets—Feminor Sequential; Orthonovin-SQ; Sequens.

2 Progestins

Progesterone (figure 15) is produced by the corpus luteum, the placenta and, in minute quantities, by the adrenal cortex. It is the only naturally occurring progestin which is found in the peripheral blood. It is produced in much larger quantities than are the oestrogens. Up to 30 mg per day are produced by the human corpus luteum in the second half of a normal cycle and during pregnancy plasma levels range between 4 and 20 mg per 100 ml but there is a rapid turnover and the half-life of blood progesterone is only four minutes. The main urinary metabolite of progesterone is pregnanediol which accounts for 10 to 20 per cent of the ovarian output. Urinary output is low in the first half of the cycle but rises in the presence of a functional corpus luteum.

Progestational agents inhibit the pituitary secretion of gonado-trophins. Under the influence of progesterone the oestrogen-primed human endometrium increases in thickness to a maximum of 5 to 7 mm, the glands become tortuous and distended with a glycogen-rich secre-

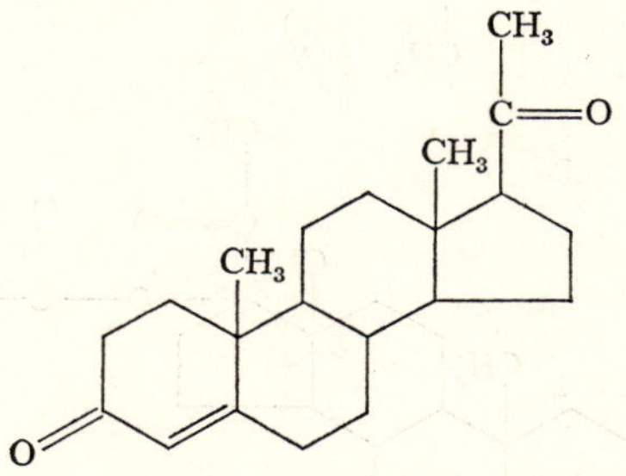

Fig. 15. Progesterone.

tion, the stroma is oedematous and the spiral arteries develop to their fullest extent. Menstruation normally occurs from an endometrium which has undergone progestational hypertrophy. Progesterone stimulates the formation of alveoli in the breast but outside the reproductive system it has fewer general effects than the oestrogens. Its metabolite, pregnanediol, causes an increase in the basal metabolic rate and is responsible for the rise in basal body temperature in the second half of an ovulatory cycle. It does not affect the blood lipids.

The actions of progesterone are modified by preceding exposure to oestrogens and in appropriate doses oestrogens and progesterone act synergistically: both the proportions and absolute amounts are important but the exact basis of this synergism is not understood.

The synthetic progestagens are more potent than progesterone, when assayed by the histological response of the oestrogen-primed endo-metrium of the ovariectomized rabbit uterus or by the endometrial content of carbonic anhydrase, although this activity is not necessarily related to the inhibition of ovulation in women. They are active orally. Progestational agents are difficult to classify and only a limited number of biological properties can be predicted from the structural formula. Three of the artificial steroids are related to 17α-hydroxyprogesterone

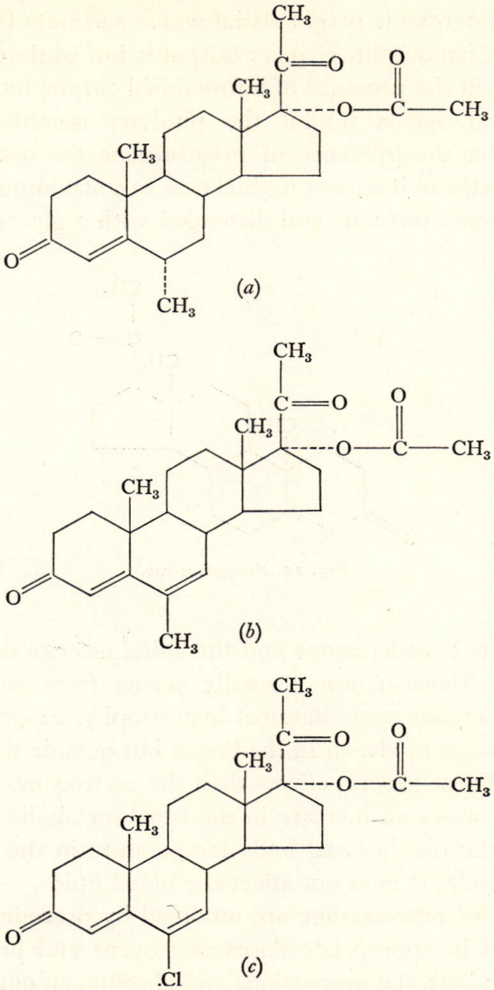

Fig. 16. Progestins derived from 17α-hydroxyprogesterone. (a) Medroxyprogesterone acetate: Combination tablets—Provest. (b) Megestrol acetate: Combination tablets—Volidan. Sequential tablets—Serial-28. (c) Cloromadinone acetate: Combination tablets—Sequens.

(figure 16). The 6-methyl and 6-chloro substitutions make these steroids very potent when given orally and they have a powerful proliferative effect on the endometrium, although their ability to inhibit ovulation is not as great. They all have a methyl group attached to carbon 19. If this methyl group is replaced by a hydrogen atom then the compound

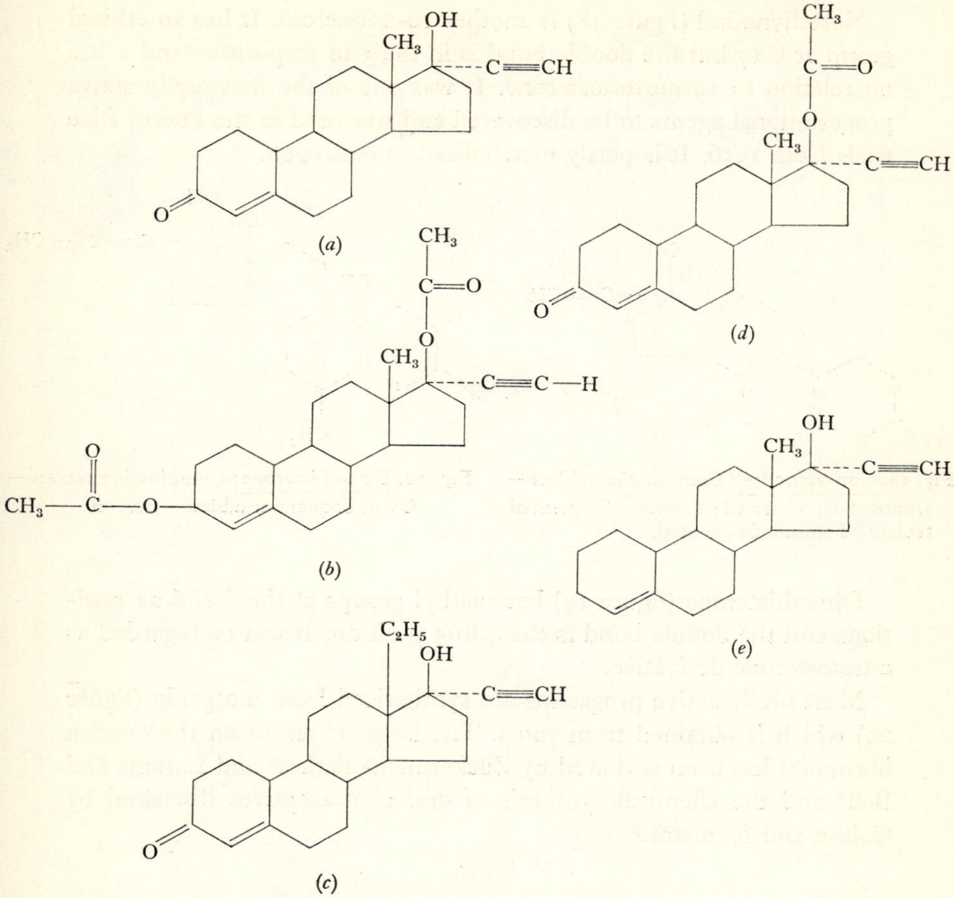

Fig. 17. 19-norsteroid progestins. (a) Norethisterone (= norethindrone): Combination tablets—Norinyl-1; Orthonovin. Sequential tablets—Orthonovin-SQ. (b) Ethynodiol diacetate: Combination tablets—Ovulen-1 mg. (c) Norgestrel: Combination tablets —Eugynon. (d) Norethisterone acetate (= norethindrone acetate): Combination tablets —Anovlar; Gynovlar-21; Norlestrin; Norlestrin-21. (e) Lynestrenol: Combination tablets—Lyndiol; Lyndiol-2·5.

is known as a 19-norsteroid. All the 19-norsteroids in use have an ethinyl group ($-C\equiv C$) at position 17. Five of them have a double bond at the 4 and 5 position (figure 17). Most of these compounds show some oestrogenic properties probably as the result of metabolism to oestrogen in the body. The double bond in the 4 and 5 position also makes them structurally analogous to 19-nortestosterone.

95

Norethynodrel (figure 18) is another 19-norsteroid. It has an ethinyl group at C17 but the double bond is in the 5 to 10 position and it has no relation to 19-nortestosterone. It was one of the first orally active progestational agents to be discovered and was used in the Puerto Rico trials from 1956. It is partly metabolized to oestrogen.

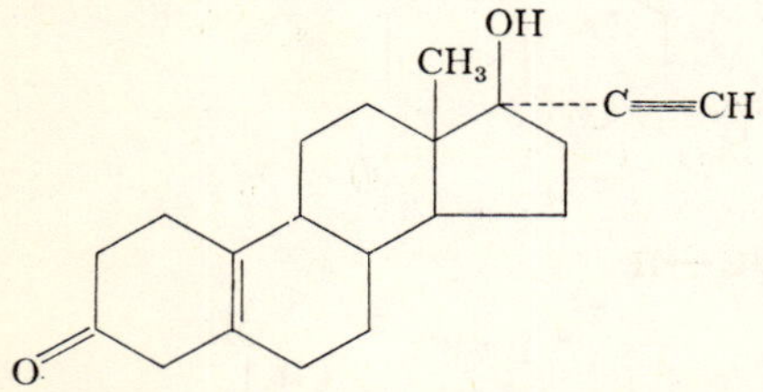

Fig. 18. Norethynodrel: Combination tablets—Conovid-E; Conovid; Enavid. Sequential tablets—Feminor Sequential.

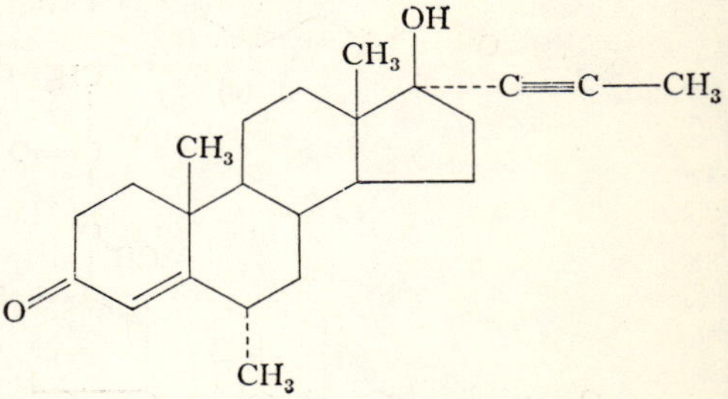

Fig. 19. Dimethisterone: Combination tablets—Ovin. Sequential tablets—Oracon.

Dimethisterone (figure 19) has methyl groups at the 6 and 21 positions and the double bond is the 4 to 5 position. It can be regarded as a testosterone derivative.

Most orally active progestins are synthesized from diosgenin (figure 20) which is obtained from yams. The large literature on the ovarian hormones has been reviewed by Zuckerman,[5] Parkes[6] and Loraine and Bell[7] and the chemical synthesis of oral contraceptives discussed by Colton and Klimstra.[8]

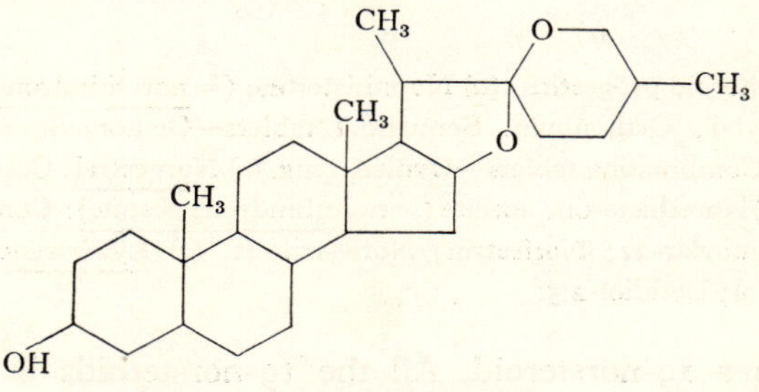

Fig. 20. Diosgenin.

Combined or serial oral contraceptives contain a progestagen and oestrogen and are taken for 20 to 22 days followed by a 6 to 8-day pause. In the sequential preparations an oestrogen is given alone for

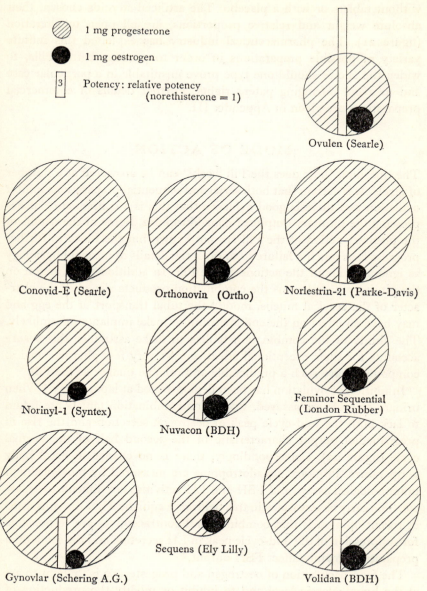

Fig. 21. Composition (monthly dose) and potency of some oral contraceptives.

14 to 16 days followed by a combined preparation and a further interval without tablets or with a placebo. The artificial steroids chosen, their absolute weight and relative proportions, are all open to alteration (figure 21). The pharmaceutical industry has exploited this infinite variety of possible preparations in order to produce better Pills, to widen the choice should one type prove unsuitable in a particular case and to avoid infringing patent rights. Further details of commercial preparations are given in Appendix III.

MODE OF ACTION

The question, 'how does the Pill work?' can be answered at a number of levels. It is certain that both serial and sequential preparations inhibit ovulation and there is good evidence that this is a consequence of depressing the pituitary output of gonadotrophins. Some of the details of the pituitary action of the Pill are not known but the block to further progress is as much a failure to unravel the details of normal physiology as ignorance about the actions of the Pill. In addition to its action on the pituitary-ovarian axis the combination products also alter the character of the cervical mucus, modify the tubal transport of the egg and may have an effect on the endometrium to make implantation unlikely. The ability of the combination tablets to make assurance thrice sure accounts for their exceptional effectiveness: very few pharmacological compounds have such a predictable and reliable quality as the Pill.

Inhibition of ovulation has been demonstrated at laporotomy.[3] When urinary steroids are assayed, women on combination tablets are found to lack both the mid-cycle peak of oestrogen secretion and the rise in pregnanediol output characteristic of the second half of the normal cycle (figure 22). Correspondingly, there is no change in basal body temperature. Pituitary gonadotrophins are measured by biological and immunological assays and FSH and LH activities are difficult to separate. The early observations in this field were equivocal but the consensus of recent opinion is that combined oral contraceptives are responsible for suppression of the mid-cycle peak in LH secretion and the sequential preparations mainly affect FSH output.[9]

The feed-back action of oestrogen and progesterone is thought to act at the hypothalamic level and to inhibit or modify the production of releasing factors for luteinizing and follicle-stimulating hormones and a hypothalamic prolactin-inhibiting factor. Oral contraceptives could have a direct effect on the ovary and several experiments have been carried out to test the ovarian responsiveness to exogenous gonadotrophins in the presence of progestins and oestrogens: on balance, the evidence is that the artificial steroids do not affect the ovary.

Among women who have been followed over a considerable number of cycles breakthrough ovulations occur in 2 to 10 per cent of cycles. In these cases the action of the combined preparations on the other

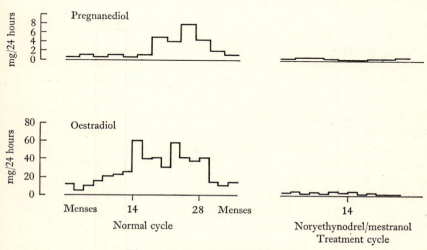

Fig. 22. Hormone excretion in urine.

links in the reproductive chain is important. Enavid, for example, renders the cervical mucus hostile to sperm.[10] Norethynodrel alone will prevent implantation in the rat when given during the first five days of pregnancy although, in physiological doses, it does not interrupt pregnancy after implantation has taken place[11] and it seems likely that the uterine epithelium of a woman taking a serial oral contraceptive is also unsuitable for receiving the fertilized egg even if ovulation and fertilization have taken place. The sequential preparations produce less alteration in endometrial histology and cervical mucus which may account for differences when failure rates are compared with those of the combined tablets.

Detailed reviews of the mode of action of oral contraceptives are provided by Mears,[12] Drill,[13] and Pincus.[14]

EFFECTIVENESS

Oral contraceptives are widely used by women of every social stratum in both developed and underdeveloped countries (figure 25). The Pill is the only method of contraception which is to all intents and purposes

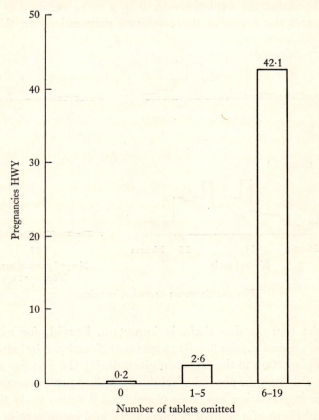

Fig. 23. Pregnancy rate following tablet omission (norethynodrel/mestranol) Enavid 5 mg.

completely effective. Drill[13] has summarized the published data on Enavid and found a total pregnancy rate, due to both patient and tablet failure, of 0·028 per HWY among 14,840 women over 116,000 cycles. Only among the small group of women who constitute problem families has a failure rate approaching that of any other method been found. Most failures are due to incorrect use and on average tablets are incorrectly taken in about 1 in 10 cycles. In about half these cases the forgotten tablet is made good later but in the remainder one or more tablets are omitted altogether. The risk of pregnancy rises with the number of tablets missed (figure 23). Errors in tablet-taking appear to be more serious in the case of sequential preparations and published series demonstrate a pregnancy rate between 1·2 and 7·1 per HWY. However, it must be emphasized that it is statistically very difficult to compare two methods of contraception if they are both highly effective (p. 41).

CLINICAL SIDE EFFECTS

In 1959 Pincus and his co-workers carried out small-scale Pill trials with three groups of women who continued with conventional contraceptives over the first few cycles: one group was given a placebo and the other two oral contraceptives, one with and one without warning of possible side effects.[15] Those who had the Pill without prior explanation had the least side effects (6·3 per cent) while those on the placebo or receiving the Pill knowing about possible complications had most complaints (17·1 and 23·3 per cent respectively) and were statistically indistinguishable. The ethical and practical difficulties of conducting further trials of the Pill involving placebos are formidable and today nearly all women are well briefed in the possible side effects. An innocuous placebo can have a powerful effect and emotional factors are likely to be particularly important in the field of contraception. It has been established that the incidence of nausea is highest in women who consider themselves emotionally tense. The incidence of side effects recorded for the same product differs widely in various trials (table 5).

TABLE 5. *Range of incidence of side effects reported by different authors for same preparation (Anovlar)*

	Lowest %	Highest %
First-cycle nausea	1·2	25
Breast discomfort	1·8	13
Weight gain (3 lb)	1·5	54
Spotting	3·0	17
Breakthrough bleeding	2·1	5·2
Amenorrhea	0·8	3·6

Oral contraceptives are taken for longer, more regularly and by a larger number of people than almost any other drugs. It is important to know the incidence of common conditions, such as headache, and rare diseases, such as pulmonary embolus, before assessing possible side effects of the Pill. Unfortunately, this is the point where knowledge is often weakest. Statistics concerning what happens to women taking the Pill are of no consequence if nothing is known about their sisters who are not taking oral contraceptives.

In the following discussion the side effects of the Pill have been grouped into therapeutically useful, or of little significance—although it should be noted that the same compound may produce opposite effects in different groups of women. Thrombosis, which is the only proven dangerous side effect, is treated separately.

1 Useful side effects

(a) RELIEF OF DYSMENORRHEA

Dysmenorrhea is colicky pain felt over the lower abdomen, or the inside of the thighs (with or without backache), and occurs with varying degrees of nausea and faintness. It can begin before, or coincide with, the onset of bleeding and the woman may feel very ill and much disabled. Forty-five per cent of women have pain with their periods and in 12 per cent of these, the pain is severe. There is a negative correlation with parity and age and dysmenorrhea is rarely encountered in anovulatory cycles. The cyclical hormone preparations abolish dysmenorrhea in 60 to 90 per cent of cases and relieve symptoms in most of the rest.[14]

Cramping can be abdominal, like a stitch, or in the calves but unlike dysmenorrhea the woman does not feel ill. The incidence of cramping can be slightly increased by oral contraceptives, especially in the initial cycles of use.

(b) RELIEF OF PREMENSTRUAL TENSION

Premenstrual tension usually lasts for three or four days but sometimes up to ten days and may end 24 hours before the onset of the menses. There is depression, with an inability to concentrate and perhaps episodes of crying, together with irritability characterized by a variation in mood and emotional outbursts. The woman may feel bloated, especially over the lower abdomen and breasts, and headaches, migraine and some forms of epilepsy are more common premenstrually. About a third of normal women complain of premenstrual irritability, a quarter of depression, anxiety, or reduction in physical activity and for many life is appreciably disturbed. Dalton has shown that there is a relation between phases of the menstrual cycle and numerous activities, such as examination performance, and over half the fatal accidents to fertile women occur during menstruation or the four days preceding it.[16] Most intellectual and motor functions are depressed premenstrually, and suicide and hospital admission for psychiatric indications are increased.

Nearly every woman is familiar with the concept of premenstrual tension and there is general agreement that oral contraceptives alleviate the symptoms much more commonly than they aggravate or induce them[17] (table 6).

TABLE 6. *Effect of oral contraceptives (ethynodiol acetate 0·5 mg with mestranol 0·1 mg) on premenstrual syndrome*

| | (Number patients, 48) Incidence (%) | |
Symptom	Before oral contraceptive	After 3 cycles of oral contraceptive
Irritability	52	2
Depression	28	8
Breast discomfort	28	14

(c) MENSTRUATION

Menstruation is largely a product of civilized living. The primitive condition is for women to be pregnant or lactating during most of their reproductive lives and the importance given to periodic bleeding in the modern world is a reflection of the desire to control fertility: menstruation tells a woman she is not pregnant but at the same time reassures her about her future fertility. The cyclical administration of the Pill mimics menstruation in a convincing way (in the case of combined products the bleeding is physiologically unlike normal menstruation) and produces some welcome improvements in what is normally a slightly messy phenomenon. Women on oral contraceptives have raised haemoglobin levels, partly as a result of decreased menstrual loss.[18]

The first generation of oral contraceptives were made up in 20s, 21s and 22s, and the first tablet in each packet was related to the beginning of the preceding menses and not to the end of the previous series of pills. As withdrawal bleeding usually follows within two or three days of finishing a packet less than 5 per cent of cycles fell outside the normal range. Today, practically all Pills are packaged to be taken seven days after ending the preceding series (regardless of the exact onset of bleeding) which has brought menstruation a clockwork predictability and eliminated some of the problems of Pill taking which arose when bleeding was slight or non-existent.

Fifty per cent or more of the women taking combined products have some reduction in loss. Less than one in twenty report an increased loss but some of this group are women who previously had abnormally scanty periods. The sequential method produces endometrial changes which are histologically similar to those of the normal cycle and not surprisingly more women using this method report unchanged, or increased, loss than those using combined products. Menstrual changes due to the Pill generally take some cycles to become fully established.

A reduction in menstrual flow should be socially and economically welcome. However, certain groups of women have mythologized menstruation, believing it to be beneficial in ridding the body of dangerous poisons. A bright red loss is associated with health and may be described as 'pretty' whereas a light loss will be considered 'bad' and reassurance and explanation may be needed.

A small group of women fail to have a period within seven days of stopping a course of tablets. This is called missed menstruation and occurs in 1 per cent or less of cycles, but up to one-fifth of women on the Pill may experience missed menstruation at some time. The condition is not significant and Mears[12] records the case of a patient in whom amenorrhea persisted for 12 months and eventually it was felt that the condition should be explored but as soon as medication was discontinued the woman became pregnant.

Changes in the pattern of menstruation are easy to quantify and Drill[13] has reviewed the literature in detail.

(d) RELIEF OF ACNE

Acne is an inflammation of sebaceous glands, probably in response to the escape of sebum into the follicular wall. The secretion of sebum is primarily controlled by androgens and the rise in ovarian androgens which occurs at puberty is responsible for female acne. Acne improves in 80 to 90 per cent of women on either combined or sequential preparations, although it may take two or three cycles for the improvement to take place.[19] In a very small number of women (less than 1 per cent) acne is aggravated by the use of the Pill.

(e) RELIEF OF HIRSUTISM

Some types of hirsutism are associated with raised serum testosterone and androstenedione levels and in these cases oral contraceptives are sometimes beneficial.

(f) RELIEF OF MITTELSCHMERZ

Pain at ovulation, lasting from a few hours or up to a day or more, is much rarer than pain at menstruation. Some women require bed rest or symptomatic treatment and others have soreness and dyspareunia. It is, of course, eliminated by both combined and sequential preparations.

(g) LIBIDO

Even if libido could be quantified there is no satisfactory information about changes in the sexual appetite at different times of life and among different women. In the first report on Enavid Pincus found that coital frequency rose in 50 per cent and fell in 40 per cent of women after beginning oral contraception.[15]

(h) WELL-BEING

The majority of couples feel that their overall 'life situation' improves after beginning oral contraceptives and in many the benefits are profound and far reaching. Among nearly 200 women treated in general practice, Murphy[20] found that the average number of surgery attendances dropped from 4·8 per year before receiving oral contraceptives to 1·8 afterwards. He compared the 'alert, jolly, and bright-eyed woman calling for her repeat prescription of oral contraceptive' with the 'anxious, sullen-faced drab who, perhaps as little as six months previously, had ...asked in hopeless tones, as an aside from her myriad complaints, for information on the Pill'.

2 Trivial or annoying side effects

(a) WEIGHT GAIN

Five to 50 per cent of women on oral contraceptives gain weight.[14] The tendency to put on weight is greatest in the first six months of use.

Often the increase in weight is trivial and sometimes it is limited to fluid retention.

Possible actions of oral contraceptives on glucose metabolism are discussed below (p. 113).

(b) BREASTS

The breasts respond to circulating oestrogen and progesterone and in normal cycles some discomfort preceding menstruation is reported by about one in six women. Engorgement and fullness appear to be a response to progesterone; pain, soreness, tenderness to oestrogen. Oral contraceptives expose the breasts to a slightly different hormonal environment and whereas some of the women who previously had breast discomfort are relieved (table 6), in others the symptoms may appear for the first time. Discomfort is virtually absent when women start oral contraceptives soon after delivery.

The Pill can be associated with some breast enlargement, but Rubens appears to have a certain long-term popularity and women rarely complain of an increase in the bust measurement.

(c) HEADACHE AND MIGRAINE

Little is known about the incidence of headaches in the normal population and complaints concerning headaches amongst Pill users should be evaluated critically. An attempt has been made to relate the incidence of headaches to arteriolar changes in the endometrium but as neither parameter can be qualified and no controls were used the results are of questionable value and it is notable that, whatever changes that do occur in the endometrium, they are not reflected in the retinal vessels.[21]

In a small group of women the Pill appears to induce headaches, especially during the interval when tablets are not being taken, and when this happens the symptom may persist over many cycles and prove resistant to changes in preparation. Migraine may be reactivated, or precipitated for the first time, by oral contraceptives.

(d) ALOPECIA

Alopecia has been reported in oral contraceptive users, but in trials of Enavid only 5 per cent of those on the drug, against 8 per cent of a control group, complained of hair loss while 6 per cent of those taking the drug alleged an arrest of previous hair loss.[14]

(e) HYPERTROPHIC GINGIVITIS

Hypertrophy of the tissue around the necks of the teeth is a recognized complication of pregnancy and may also occur in women taking oral progestagens.[22] In extreme cases an epulis may form, although more commonly the gums may be sore or the hypertrophied tissue become the site of infections such as Vincent's disease and pyorrhea. The condition is usually remedied by good oral hygiene.

(f) CORNEAL OEDEMA

Some women are less tolerant of contact lenses premenstrually and oral contraceptives have also been reported to make contact lenses more difficult to use in a small number of patients. If the lenses are used for cosmetic, and not for opthalmological, indications the patient must choose between her face and her fertility. Very rarely the oedema is severe and could lead to corneal scarring in which case oral contraceptives must be prohibited.

There is no reliable evidence linking oral contraceptives with any other eye diseases and they are not contraindicated in glaucoma.

(g) VAGINAL DISCHARGE

Mucorrhoea is associated with high plasma oestrogen levels and may occur in some women on oral contraceptives. In a few cases the Pill aggravates or precipitates moniliasis. Active treatment is necessary for what can be a very trying condition.

(h) MISCELLANEOUS

As up to one-third of the fertile women in a population may be taking the Pill a large number of fortuitous relationships occur between this form of contraception and various diseases. Possibly oral contraceptives can precipitate episodes of eczema and urticaria but remission, as well as a worsening, has been reported where the condition existed before the Pill was given. Arthralgia and myalgia have been reported in Pill users but these entities are too vague to permit meaningful comment.

Some women are aware of the hormonal changes characteristic of pregnancy at a very early stage. These same women may experience similar changes when on the Pill—so much so that they may think it has failed.

3   Thrombo-embolic phenomena

Deep vein thrombosis is a condition which is peculiarly difficult to diagnose. There may be unilateral swelling, especially of the calf, although venous anastomoses cut down the significance of this sign. Pain is often absent even on pressure over the affected vein, or on dorsiflexion of the foot, and the condition may be totally silent. Clinical findings and postmortem observations agree only in a minority of cases and careful observers miss two-thirds of cases while, conversely, experienced surgeons diagnose deep vein thrombosis in twice as many cases as it can be demonstrated by phlebography.

When the diagnosis is so unsure any statistics regarding venous thrombosis must be handled carefully. Apparently dramatic associations may be coincidental and most of the comments which litter the medical journals by individual doctors about what their patients did or did not do on the Pill are meaningless. The possibility of making false associations is well illustrated by the doctor who gave a woman a prescription for Enavid and six weeks later found she had an episode of thrombophlebitis; only on further investigation was it discovered that she had failed to have the prescription dispensed. Only large series with adequate controls provide valid information.

The balance of hormones found during pregnancy appears to protect against thrombophlebitis and in reviewing the world literature Drill[13] found a rate of 0·73 cases per 1,000 women-pregnancies per year against 1·2 to 2·9 cases of 1,000 non-pregnant women. Post-partum thrombophlebitis and embolic phenomena run at the much higher rate of between 3·1 and 10·4 cases per 1,000 deliveries.

The first report in the British literature of a thrombotic episode in a woman on oral contraceptives was made in 1961.[23] As far as is known, thrombosis is the potentially most dangerous complication of oral contraception and it is unfortunate that appraisal of the subject is bedevilled by the statistical difficulties of dealing with rare events, the problems of accurate diagnosis and reporting, and ignorance of the full details of normal blood clotting.

The American Food and Drug Administration (1963)[24] surveyed deaths due to thrombo-embolic phenomena among users of Enavid and estimated a death rate of 12·1 per million against 8·4 in control women and concluded that there was no significant difference. The British Committee on Safety of Drugs published a preliminary report in 1967

TABLE 7. *Thrombo-embolism in women on the Pill*

Cause of death (patients with no predisposing condition)	Number	Number using oral contraceptives		Statistical significance
		Actual	Predicted	
Pulmonary embolism	26	16	4·2	$P<0·001$
Coronary thrombosis	84	18	11·4	$P<0·06$
Cerebral thrombosis	10	5	1·5	$P<0·01$

and concluded that 'there can be no reasonable doubt that some types of thrombo-embolic disorder are associated with use of oral contraceptives'.[25] The negative results in the earlier studies probably arose because some doctors were unwilling to report side effects in a drug they used widely and favoured greatly. It is possible, although less likely, that geographical or ethnic differences control the response of a population to oral contraceptives.

Two important papers from the British Committee on the Safety of Drugs and the Medical Research Council in 1968 confirm the risk of thrombo-embolic phenomena and allow a fairly accurate assessment of morbidity and mortality.[26,27] Among 499 women age 20 to 44, whose deaths were certified as due to pulmonary, cerebral or coronary thrombosis or embolism, 309 were married women in a situation unassociated with any other fatal disease and with the possibility of adequate follow-up. When compared with a control group of 988 women, selected from the records of doctors who had care of the fatal cases, a significantly increased number of oral contraceptive users was found among those dying of pulmonary embolism and cerebral thrombosis and possibly also in the case of coronary thrombosis (table 7). It is important to note that the majority of the diagnoses were substantiated by post mortems and bias in the case of the fatal cases seems unlikely. The overall mortality attributed to oral contraceptives is calculated as 1·3 per 100,000 in the 20 to 34 age-group and 3·4 in the 35 to 44 age-group. There are reasons for thinking that this may underestimate the total death rate and if relationship between coronary thrombosis and the Pill is substantiated the figures will be 2·2 and 4·5 respectively. Among 58 patients admitted to hospital with deep vein thrombosis or pulmonary embolism, but without any predisposing disease, 26 (45 per cent) were found to be using oral contraceptives in the month before admission. In a control group only 9 per cent of women had been using oral contraceptives. There are reasons to believe that the doctors referring the patients to hospital were not unduly biased by a lively awareness that thrombosis might be associated with the Pill. The use of oral contraceptives probably causes a ninefold rise in the risk of being admitted to hospital with venous thrombo-embolism, or put another way approximately 1 woman in every 2,000 using oral contraceptives will be admitted to hospital yearly.

The evidence linking thrombo-embolism and oral contraceptives does not suggest that any particular parity group is at risk, or that any preparation is more or less dangerous, but there are more deaths among women over 35 years of age. Fat women are more prone to suffer thrombotic episodes and on average Pill users gain weight, but the available evidence is too limited to decide if these effects overlap, sum or act synergistically. A history of thrombo-embolism predisposes to recurrence but it is difficult to compute the added risk with oral contraceptives and it must be remembered that the risks of thrombo-embolism in pregnancy will also be increased.

Blood clotting is one of the most complex physiological processes involving platelets, tissue damage, surface contact and a number of clotting factors which may be pre-enzymes activated by other enzymes. In addition there are a number of inhibiting factors which destroy any activated factor within a few minutes of formation. Blood clotting remains incompletely understood and the significance of tests designed to quantify particular steps in the process is difficult to assess. Oral contraceptives bring about a reduction in clotting time but leave the bleeding time unaltered. When individual factors are measured, mean prothrombin time decreases and fibrinogen concentration, fibrinolytic activity, factor VII and factor VIII increase.[14]

The changes are thought to be oestrogen dependent, and preparations with low oestrogen dosage may carry less risk. If progestagens alone could be made into an acceptable contraceptive there would be no risk of inducing thrombosis.

ORAL CONTRACEPTIVES AND
NORMAL PHYSIOLOGY

1 Central nervous system and pituitary

The histology of the pituitary gland in women using oral contraceptives is practically unknown and it will take many years to answer even some of the questions that might be asked. In rats an increase in chromophobe tissue has been reported in one long-term study of norethynodrel but the changes were not clear cut.[28] No alteration in pituitary weight has been reported in monkeys on oral contraceptives.[29] In a report from Australia Shearman found 9 out of 86 patients with secondary amenorrhea had previously used oral contraceptives.[30] The ovaries responded to exogenous gonadotrophins and the failure appeared to be at the hypothalamic or pituitary level. However, a larger series needs to be investigated as up to one-third of married women in Australia take the Pill.

The rapid return of normal pituitary function after a course of oral contraceptives suggests that long-term damage is unlikely. The ability of the pituitary to recover from a long period of depression is well illustrated by the case of a woman who had an adrenal tumour secreting large quantities of progesterone which had caused 20 years of amenorrhea. One month after surgical removal she had a normal period and continued to menstruate until the menopause.

There is no evidence that oral contraceptives alter pituitary function at puberty or the menopause, although fuller evidence concerning the effect of exogenous steroids in the early years after the menarche would be useful. As oestrogens promote closure of the epiphyses they could prevent a young girl reaching her full stature.

2 Genital tract

The ovaries of women using oral contraceptives appear macroscopically like those of a post-menopausal woman and, with rare exceptions, lack corpora lutea. Histologically there are no mature follicles and the tunica may be thickened; however, the ovarian response to gonadotrophin stimulation appears unchanged.[31]

Oral contraceptives may affect tubal motility. With combination tablets the endometrial glands are rapidly transformed through the proliferative phase so that the secretory phase, normally fully developed by days 19 to 20, occurs within a few days of commencing the tablets.

The endometrium is hypoplastic and pseudodecidual changes occur in the stromal tissue. With sequential therapy a proliferative endometrium is found with the unopposed oestrogens, secretory changes are delayed until the progestagen is added, the endometrium remains active and pseudodecidual changes do not occur. There is a rapid return to full histological normality, including fine structure, at the cessation of treatment.

Uterine fibromyomata may enlarge during oral contraceptive therapy but they are a common entity and no controlled observations have been made on the subject. Cervical erosions are thought to be more common, at least on combined regimes, but there is no association with atypical smears and the condition regresses with the cessation of oral contraceptives.

3   Adrenal

Prolonged administration of norsteroids have no effect on adrenal histology but the oestrogens in oral contraceptives do cause an increase in transcortin (corticosteroid-binding globulin) which leads to a raised total aldosterone.[32] This appears to be unassociated with any increase in aldosterone output although it may be responsible for changes in plasma pyruvate.

4   Thyroid

As in the case of the adrenal, there is a change in plasma carriage and thyroxine-binding globulin rises when oral contraceptives are given and as a consequence the protein-bound iodine increases from approximately 5 μg to 7–8 μg per 100 ml.[14] This change is independent of dosage, is not progressive, returns to normal when the tablets are discontinued and has no demonstrable effect on overal physiology as the radiothyroid uptake is unaltered.

Changes in the protein-bound iodine can lead to the misinterpretation of clinical tests of thyroid function. Radio-iodine uptake and excretion give valid results in women on oral contraceptives but the resin uptake of labelled triiodothyronine and protein-bound iodine tests should not be measured on anyone who has used oral contraceptives within the past six weeks.

5   Liver

Empirical tests of liver function are difficult to interpret and the most useful studies include pretreatment controls.

The liver is the main source of serum proteins, with the exception of the α-globulins which are produced in the reticulo-endothelial system. The cephalin flocculation and thymol turbidity tests, which reflect any imbalance in the serum proteins and the serum bilirubin and alkaline phosphatase levels, which rise in biliary obstruction and hepatocellular damage, are all unaffected by oral contraceptives.[14,33] Abnormal serum transaminase readings, which are elevated when there is cell damage, have been found by some workers. In Britain and the United States no statistical difference has been detected between controls and oral contraceptive users, but 4 to 6 per cent abnormal readings have been found in Scandinavia.[34] It remains to be established whether these divergent results are due to ethnic or to experimental differences. Raised bromsulphalein (BSP) retention tests have also been found in some women on the Pill. The test is a measure of the hepatic ability to concentrate a dye and excrete it into the bile, which rises during pregnancy and in response to exogenous oestrogens. Allan and Tyler[35] found 2·3 per cent of a control group and 6·8 per cent of Pill users ($P < 0.05$) had abnormal (10 per cent or more after 45 min) BSP retention tests. The percentage of abnormals declined as the length of time since starting the tablets increased; low dosage preparations produced fewest abnormals and 1 mg norethisterone was without any demonstrable effect. Obese women and those in the luteal phase of the normal cycle also tend to have a prolonged BSP retention.

6 Metabolic

In some women the response to a glucose tolerance test varies with the stage of the menstrual cycle, being greatest when circulating oestrogens are lowest.

Abnormal glucose tolerance tests have been reported in 18 to 46 per cent of women taking oral contraceptives. The variation arises partly from the use of differing criteria and partly from the lack of adequate controls. Wynn and Doar[36] studied 105 non-diabetic women on combined oral contraceptives and compared them with 78 controls matched for age, parity and body weight. A statistically significant decline in oral and intravenous glucose tolerance was found in the test group. It is difficult to interpret tests which differ only slightly from normal. In some ways, the changes described by Wynn and Doar resemble those taking place in pregnancy. Pregnancy diabetes is often a precursor of frank diabetes but unfortunately the physiological basis of the condition is unknown. It may be significant that the incidence of abnormal tests in oral contraceptive users is greatest in women with a family history of diabetes. Careful prospective studies of women using oral contraceptives over several years are needed.

Wynn and Doar also found that women on oral contraceptives also show changes in the serum triglyceride, cholesterol, low-density and very-low-density lipoproteins which are all raised.[37]

ORAL CONTRACEPTIVES AND SUBSEQUENT FERTILITY

There is some evidence that the withdrawal of norethynodrel from animals is followed by a rebound increase in fertility and there have been hints of a parallel phenomenon in the literature relating to human fertility after ceasing to use oral contraceptives. In the British CIFC trial 80 per cent of women became pregnant within two months of stopping the Pill. However, it seems likely that, in any population, the first group who choose to use an oral contraceptive includes many women of above average fecundity who bias the results.

The largest follow-up series available is of 240 pregnancies among Puerto Rican women who stopped using Enavid after one to six years.[38] Ninety per cent of the women conceived within two months and it is certain that oral contraceptives have no general effect on subsequent fertility. It would, of course, be very difficult to detect rare and idiosyncratic changes in fertility unless a much larger series were used, and even then it would be difficult to sort the consequential from the co-incidental.

ORAL CONTRACEPTION AND FETAL ABNORMALITY

There is no statistical evidence of any increase in the incidence of congenital abnormalities in babies born to women who have been on oral contraceptives. Nevertheless, some discussion is necessary to deal with biologically tenable, if unsubstantiated, fears.

It has been claimed that high doses (10 mg or more) of orally acting norsteroids, when given for obstetric indications, may be associated with female virilization.[39] The evidence is weak and there is no reason to think that it applies to the use of oral contraceptives.

Permanent sterility and marked behavioural changes can be produced in newborn rats by the administration of a variety of steroid hormones, either given directly or through the lactating mother.[40] It is probable that there is a stage in all mammals when the brain is particularly sensitive to circulating hormones and can be 'switched' to a new pattern of behaviour, although the timing of this event may show marked species differences. If this hypothetical danger is ever confirmed then the use of hormones for obstetrical reasons or to suppress lactation will present a graver risk than the Pill, if only because the concurrent use of oral contraceptives and pregnancy is exceptionally rare.

In a small series of eight abortuses from women who had become pregnant after stopping oral contraceptives Carr[41] found four triploid/diploid mosaics against only 23 in 521 controls. Two XO (Turner's syndrome) fetuses were also found in the same series. A triploid number of chromosomes is incompatible with survival and only one in 40 Turner's syndrome survive to birth. Variations in steroid hormones in the cycle following oral contraceptives might cause delay in tubal transport of the egg which in turn could predispose to triploidy. A larger series is necessary and if a relation with the Pill is substantiated then it would become necessary to recommend the use of a mechanical form of contraception in the first few cycles after discontinuing the oral contraceptives. A parallel risk might apply to couples using the rhythm method, who avoid intercourse at the estimated time of ovulation.

The WHO Report on oral contraception[42] suggests that a five-year follow-up study of at least 10,000 children born to women who have taken the Pill, should be undertaken, including investigation of the sex ratio and twinning frequency.

ORAL CONTRACEPTIVES AND MALIGNANCY

Cancerphobias are common in Western societies and many patients want to discuss the possible carcinogenic effects of oral contraceptives. Certain malignancies, especially mammary cancer, are known to be partially dependent on the sex hormones. Known carcinogens, such as shale oil, X-rays and radioactive ores, have a latent period of 5 to 30 years in man and it can be argued that adverse effects from oral contraceptives have not yet had time to appear.

The absolute dose of hormone given, the ratio of oestrogen and progesterone, the length of time given and the species of animal under consideration are all important in evaluating data relating cancer to steroid hormones. The most relevant information comes from the human field. In women receiving exogenous oestrogen for long periods no increase in the incidence of cancer has been noted. For example, among 304 patients receiving oestrogen for an average of seven to eight years each, there were no cases of ovarian, cervical, uterine or breast carcinoma although in a normal population 18 cases would be expected.[43] Among over 1,000 women receiving massive doses of oestrogen for inoperable breast cancer no endometrial primaries were found.[44]

There have been no reports of an increased incidence of any form of cancer among the millions of women on the Pill. Up to 1967 the FDA files contain only one record of cancer of the breast in a woman on oral contraceptives. Cervical cancer and precancerous states have been particularly closely studied because of the habit of taking Papanicolaou smears. Rice-Wray and her co-workers[45] studied 2,040 women over 22,948 cycles on Enavid and found no positive smears on annual cervical examination, although they predicted 11·8 positive smears from study of the normal population. But current studies in the United States suggest an opposite result. When Pill and diaphragm users are matched for several parameters the former have a higher incidence of suspicious smears and (when biopsies are carried out) of carcinoma in situ. Reviewing the evidence available at the end of 1968, the Medical Committee of the International Planned Parenthood Federation concluded[46] that a causal relationship could be neither established nor refuted and that the benefits of the Pill outweigh all possible hazards. At the same time it emphasized the wisdom of annual smears and suggested that available cytological services should be extended. The full findings of the current studies will be eagerly awaited, although a great deal more work will be required to establish the true nature of any possible relationship and to assess the magnitude of the risk if it is present. When regular cervical smears are obtained abnormal cells and carcinoma in situ can be treated and, unlike thrombo-embolic conditions, they are virtually one hundred per cent curable.

PRESCRIBING

1 General

There is no doubt that oral contraceptives are the most effective and widely acceptable contraceptive now available. The number of women who give up the Pill because of adverse side effects is probably less than those who abandon it for irrational reasons. Absolute contra-indications to its use are exceedingly rare although there are several instances where caution may be needed.

The doctor prescribing the Pill must be alert to the problems which worry women concerning oral contraceptives and willing to answer the unspoken as well as the overt questions. In lower social groups questions are based either on the folklore which surrounds human reproduction or arise from dullness of comprehension. In educated women the questions are more likely to be of the sort that the woman is suspicious of upsetting her 'hormonal balance'. Objections to taking the Pill can be deep-seated and unexpected, as in a patient of the author's who refused the Pill because she was a vegetarian and thought it was made from animal hormones—she took it with alacrity when told it was manufactured from yams.

The husband or boy friend is an important factor in a woman's attitudes to contraception, particularly in lower social groups where the phrase 'my husband won't let me take the Pill' is common. Unfortunately labourers or mechanics are less likely to come and discuss their reservations with a doctor than are solicitors or bank clerks, but a great deal can be done to answer a husband's questions by face-to-face interview or through the embassy of the wife. There is an almost universal awareness that dangerous side effects have been reported in women taking the Pill. Thrombosis is widely known, and can only be answered by fitting the risk into the context of the dangers which everyone is forced to take in their daily life. The fear of cancer and danger of fetal damage is a persistent one. This latter fear is particularly well marked in some groups such as immigrants. The magnitude of lay misunderstanding of the Pill is brought out by the fact that some people think oral contraceptives are synonymous with thalidomide.

Present-day oral contraceptives are packaged either in tear-off foil strips, punch-out plastic mounts or in dial packs. Most presentations include a method of specifying the day of the week so the patient must start at a particular point in the series and work round until all the tablets have been taken. Packets have simple, clear instructions printed on them. Some packs provide a space for entering the date and clinics may provide calendars where tablets, periods and even coitus are entered, but few people persist with these records after the first cycle.

Most women find no difficulty in taking the Pill. It is easiest to remember the tablets if some regular time of day is chosen to take them. The patient must be instructed to:

1. Count the first day of her next period as DAY 1.

2. Take the first tablet of her first cycle on DAY 5, whether or not her menstrual loss has ceased.

3. Take one tablet daily until the packet is completed. In the case of sequential regimes she will be faced with tablets of different colours.

4. If she forgets a tablet she must take it as soon as she remembers the omission and the next day's tablet should be taken at the normal time: this usually means she will have missed one day and taken two tablets in the course of the next day.

5. At the end of the course she must, according to the preparation used, either

(a) wait until bleeding commences and begin the next packet on DAY 5 and if no bleeding occurs begin the next packet on DAY 7, or

(b) wait SEVEN days and begin the next packet regardless of the time of onset of menstruation.

6. If breakthrough bleeding occurs (see below) the woman should continue the medication. If a full period occurs she should stop taking the tablets and begin the next packet five days after the bleeding began.

The system of 21 tablets followed by a gap of seven days is now widely used and the patient always begins the Pill on the same day of the week. Some sequential regimes are made up with a placebo so the woman takes a Pill daily as long as she uses the method and the same has been done for combined preparations by adding seven oral iron tablets.

The woman is fully protected against pregnancy as soon as she takes the first tablet, except in the case of the minority who sometimes have very short cycles—21 days or less—and who may ovulate early in the first cycle of use. In these cases alternative precautions should be used for the first 14 days of the first cycle. Care must be taken when changing from one type of preparation to another, especially when changing to a preparation with lower dosage and added contraceptive precautions may be necessary.

A small percentage of women need more than usual help. Such women may be particularly forgetful or unable to grasp even the simplest instruction. Some women will remove tablets from a packet so as to produce a pattern which pleases them, or will limit their tablet taking to the days when they have intercourse, or will share their prescription with friends, neighbours and unmarried sisters or take the Pill for only one week out of four. Women of this kind need repeated, calm instruction and, in the context of domiciliary family planning service, numerous visits. The husband or boy friend may provide a suitable path to regular Pill taking but there remains a tiny residual group of women who do not have a capacity to take oral contraceptives and for whom, other considerations apart, the intrauterine device appears preferable.

Failure to replenish supplies of Pills is more common than gross errors in Pill taking. Lack of foresight, a domestic life which makes it difficult to visit the doctor, clinic or chemist, or straightforward lack of housekeeping money may make a woman miss getting a fresh supply of Pills. Once a woman is established on oral contraceptives it can be helpful to prescribe for 6 or 12-month intervals (see also p. 230).

Patients should keep Pills in a safe place. The well-known story of a daughter replacing her mother's Pills with aspirins has a basis in fact and one case of an unstable husband replacing his wife's contraceptive Pills with grandfather's digoxin occurred before the easily recognized packages were introduced. Young children and toddlers may swallow large numbers of Pills, taking them to be sweets, unless the mother keeps them beyond their reach. Fortunately, there are no toxic effects and reassurance, not gastric lavage, is indicated. In nearly 100 cases of accidental ingestion by children no ill effects were reported, except for three cases of vomiting.[47]

In exceptionally rare cases the need to begin a course of oral contraceptives at other than the usual time in the cycle may arise. A woman who is poor, has a large family and will not use any other method or the muddle-headed girl who comes for advice three days before her wedding but ten days after her period might be given a highly progestational Pill immediately. The danger of starting oral contraception later than usual in the cycle is that the woman may already be pregnant and in these cases oestrogens or norethisterone (5 mg three times a day for 7 days) may be given in order to produce withdrawal bleeding, the oral contraceptive regime being started 5 days later. If a pregnancy has been terminated oral contraception can be begun 5 days after the commencement of bleeding and the Pill can be given 6 weeks after a term delivery whether menstruation has returned or not.[48]

A routine medical examination may be performed when the Pill is first prescribed and at yearly intervals. *A cervical smear should always be taken* but the remainder of the examination will be mainly determined by the demands of preventive medicine (see p. 229).

2   Choice of preparation

Rational Pill prescribing is difficult. The exact effects of the artificial steroids are not known for all target organs, the inhibition of endogenous ovarian hormones shows individual variations and the woman's expectation of a particular compound may override her physiological response: the knowledge that her neighbour has done well on one brand may be more important than the fact that it contains a powerful progestational agent likely to aggravate her acne.

Something of the woman's own hormone balance can be discovered from the history and examination. If it is predominantly oestrogenic then the following may be present:

Irritability, tiredness and premenstrual tension.
Fluid retention, weight gain and headache.
Irregular and heavy menstruation, mucous cervical discharge and
    cervical erosion.

If progestational effects are uppermost there may be:

Breast fullness.
Acne and greasy skin and hair.
Light periods with leg and abdominal cramps.
A dry vagina and a white premenstrual discharge.

Premenstrual depression occurs in some women as the progesterone levels in the body decline. Her own account of any previous pregnancy will also give some indication of how she responds to a high level of progesterone.

In starting a woman on oral contraceptives an attempt can be made to counteract any troublesome side effects that she suffers during her own cycle.

The two oestrogens in use approximate to one another in potency. However, their effects cannot be fully predicted from the dose as some progestins, for example norethynodrel, are partly metabolized to oestrogen. The relative potencies of progestins can be assayed in a variety of ways. Greenblatt[49] has compared the daily dose necessary to delay menstruation for 20 days. In figure 21 the absolute dose of steroids given during the cycle and the relative potencies of the progestin used are compared for a number of oral contraceptives. In table 8 serial preparations are classified according to their most commonly encountered clinical effect.

TABLE 8. *Progestational and oestrogenic ratios*

Strong Progestin	
	Ovulen
Anovlar	
Anovlar 21	
	Volidan
	Lyndiol
Gynovlar	Noracyclin
Volidan	Enovid
Norlestrin	
Norlestrin 21	
Lyndiol 2·5	Conovid
Anacyclin	
Norinyl	Conovid E
Orlest	Previson
Minovlar	Ortho-novum
Orthonovin-1/80	Nuvacon
Weak	

Strong oestrogen

If a woman develops troublesome side effects then it may be worth changing to another preparation. If amenorrhea (missed menses) or very scanty periods occur, and if the woman is worried by this symptom, then a more oestrogenic preparation or a sequential formula can be tried. A raised oestrogen and reduced progesterone dosage will also relieve breast fullness but if the breasts are tender or painful the converse is true. When nausea occurs, and does not settle down in one or two cycles, a preparation with a different oestrogen (mestranol for ethynyloestradiol and vice versa) can be used. If there is persistent breakthrough bleeding a higher dosage or a more progestational formulation should be used. It is, of course, essential to watch for any complicating gynaecological factor and not confuse breakthrough bleeding with inter-menstrual bleeding. Breakthrough bleeding may also be a sign that a woman is not taking the tablets regularly. A more progestational preparation is also indicated in those few women who complain of increased menstrual loss.

When weight gain is unwelcome and continues beyond the first few cycles it is worth changing to another preparation especially if a 19-norsteroid, such as norethindrone or norethindrone acetate, is being used. On the whole low dosage preparations are least likely to cause weight gain. Attention should also be paid to the woman's diet and it should be borne in mind that relief from the fear of pregnancy can be associated with an improved appetite.

In a small number of women there appears to be a marked depression of libido and in these cases it may be worth trying a different compound or considering sequential therapy, but the physician must beware of the woman who is looking for a scapegoat for her emotional problems or has found herself in an unsatisfactory home situation.

The sequential preparations provide a useful extension to the range of oral contraceptives and may have a lower incidence of certain side effects. Some of the early preparations were associated with a relatively high failure rate and only very rarely will a woman choose to use a less effective method in order to escape a particular side effect. The amount of oestrogen is critical but adequate inhibition of ovulation appears to be effected with 0·1 mg. Sequential preparations can be useful for the woman who has predominantly progestational side effects in her normal cycle. If a woman on a combined preparation, which has a primarily progestational balance, has troublesome side effects, such as missed menses, then she may feel better on sequentials. Chloasma is also said to improve on a sequential preparation. Conversely, a woman started on sequentials may have to be changed to a combined regime because of oestrogenic symptoms such as fluid retention.

3   Oral contraception and lactation

Unhappily, in the Western world, breast feeding is an unusual phenomenon and the question of prescribing oral contraceptives to lactating mothers seldom arises. The original high dosage Pills, such as 10 mg Enavid, reduced the quantity of milk production in about half the women taking them, but the lower dosage products now in use make little significant difference (figure 24) and women on the Pill have nursed their babies for a year or more.

In a double blind trial of norethisterone 1 mg with mestranol 0·05 mg (Norinyl-1) begun the day after birth and followed for eight days, lactation was not inhibited.[50] The percentage of babies having complementary feeds rose from 3·5 per cent with a placebo to 12 per cent with the drug but weight gain in the two groups of babies was similar.

Lactating women given oral contraceptives will generally resume menstruation within two or three months of beginning medication. One case of breast enlargement in a male infant nursed by a woman on oral contraceptives has been recorded but there is no statistical evidence to relate the two events, and in any case the situation was unusual, involving a high dose Pill beginning three days after delivery. Low dose oral contraceptives can be begun at the six-week post-natal examination in the case of the woman who is breast feeding.

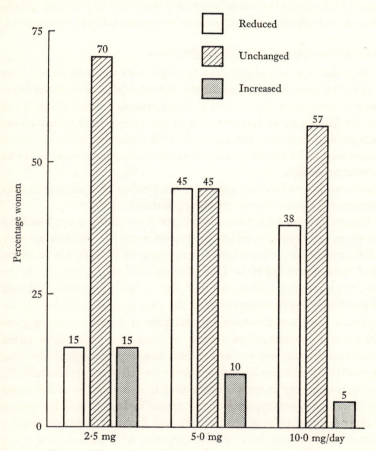

Fig. 24. Effect of norethynodrel/mestranol (Enavid) on lactation.

4 Oral contraception and puberty

The mean age of puberty has declined from approximately 17 to 12 years in the past century. No doubt this change is partly responsible for the increasingly early age at which young people are becoming sexually active. Fortunately, the need for contraceptive advice in the first four or five years after the menarche remains rare.

The consequences of interrupting pituitary activity in the first few years of adult activity is not understood and concern has occasionally been expressed about prescribing oral contraceptives for the very young. However, girls of 15 or 16 are unlikely to use any other method and the social and psychological consequences of pregnancy in the very young more than outweigh any physiological reservations which may be held.

5   Oral contraceptives and the menopause

Just as the mean age of puberty has declined over the past century, so that of the menopause is rising and the modal age is now about fifty. The factors controlling the time of the menopause are not understood but they are known to be independent of the woman's previous endocrine history and it is not, for example, influenced by the number of pregnancies earlier in life. Similarly, it is unaffected by several years of oral contraceptive use.

Oral contraceptives have no effect on the process of follicular atresia which constantly occurs in the ovaries of fertile women.[51]

Oral contraceptives have two advantages for a woman approaching the menopause: they give complete protection at an age when pregnancy is usually unwelcome, obstetrically dangerous and more likely to be associated with some types of fetal abnormality and they appear to assist in carrying some women through the difficult psychological and physiological changes that can occur at the change of life. Malignancies of the genital tract are common in menopausal women and the prescription of oral contraceptives should be used as a time when pelvic and breast examination are performed and any intermenstrual bleeding occurring after the Pill has been given must be followed up carefully.

Menstruation rarely stops abruptly and if a woman is still having regular cycles oral contraceptives can be prescribed for four or five years. If it is then decided to stop medication and discover if natural cycles recur, alternative contraceptive precaution may be recommended.

Oral contraceptives carry a greater risk of death in older women and this danger must be balanced against that of pregnancy, the risk of which rises progressively after the fifth child and is five times the overall rate by the time a tenth child is born. The doctor must attempt to assess the chance of pregnancy, the risks the pregnancy might carry, the ability of the woman to use alternative methods of contraception as well as the possible need for exogenous hormones to deal with menopausal symptoms.

6 Oral contraception and disease

Breast cancer, and any other hormone-dependent malignancy, constitutes a contra-indication to oral contraceptives. Although exogenous hormones may be useful in treatment their use demands specialist advice. Adequate contraceptive advice is, of course, of paramount importance in these cases and it is better to leave a woman on the Pill than risk a pregnancy.

Oral contraceptives are contra-indicated in women with chronic idiopathic jaundice (Dubin–Johnson and Rotor syndromes), with a past history of recurrent idiopathic jaundice of pregnancy (benign recurrent cholestatic jaundice of pregnancy), or recurrent generalized pruritis of pregnancy. These conditions are all rare, idiopathic jaundice of pregnancy, for example, occurring in 1 in 3,500 pregnancies, and they are not well understood. They are aggravated by artificial steroids.

In view of the limited effect of oral contraceptives on liver function and the ambiguity of interpreting BSP changes, a past history of infectious hepatitis should not be regarded as a contra-indication, unless liver function tests are still abnormal, when some alternative form of contraception should be advised.

Chloasma, pregnancy mask, the increased facial pigmentation which sometimes occurs in pregnancy, is a rare complication of oral contraceptives. Probably both progesterone and oestrogen are involved. Among Caucasian women it probably involves less than 1 per cent, but it was reported in up to a quarter of the women who entered the early Pill trials in Puerto Rico where many women are of Mexican extraction. It is possible to block the increase in pigmentation with vitamin B and it may be a complication of undernutrition. Oral contraceptives are inadvisable in a woman with a history of chloasma in pregnancy. Therapy may have to be discontinued if chloasma occurs for the first time when oral contraceptives are used. It is most likely in women who live in sunny climates and have been on oral contraceptives for a long time. The pigmentation may not resolve completely after treatment. Hydroquinine cream which blocks ultraviolet light may be useful.

Caution should be taken in the case of the Pill if a woman gives a history of epilepsy, multiple sclerosis, porphyria or otosclerosis, especially if the condition was aggravated by a previous pregnancy.

The more oestrogenic preparations should be avoided when there is a history of asthma.

In a number of other conditions many doctors feel uneasy about prescribing oral contraceptives but on the present evidence their caution is unjustified. None of the published series showed any relation between hypertension and the Pill. Unless fresh information becomes available there is nothing to be gained by regular sphygnomanometric records and much to be lost in worrying the patient. A family history of coronary thrombosis is common and is irrelevant when giving the Pill to women in the fertile years. When the patient gives a personal history of thrombosis, at any site, the consequences of prescribing oral contraceptives are more grave. Nevertheless, a prescription can be justified if no alternative method of family planning is acceptable, especially as pregnancy also carries an increased risk of recurrence. Varicose veins and obesity present a similar but slightly simpler situation because the risks are less. It is unwise to treat varicose veins by injection when a woman is on the Pill.

EVALUATION

Until the current generation of oral contraceptives is replaced by more advanced types their widespread use is socially imperative and more than justifiable medically. Although they are now known to carry a measurable mortality, when this risk is set against that of death due to pregnancy and delivery (see page 254) the use of oral contraceptives proves safer than nearly all the other possibilities that are open to a married woman.

Oral contraceptives are more widely acceptable than any other method and many women would take the Pill in order to obtain the effectiveness and convenience which it offers whatever the risk attached to it. The Pill has made contraceptive advice available to whole groups within society where none of the previously available methods was of the slightest use. Its impact in developing nations, as yet hardly felt, will probably prove as great as it has already been in many Western countries (figure 25).

Oral contraceptives are usually the first choice for the young woman, especially if intercourse is taking place outside marriage or if a young married couple wish to postpone having children for a number of years in order to complete some sort of training or education. They are also particularly suitable for the woman who has completed her family but who remains highly fertile.

Like all other methods of contraception the Pill can have side effects, but it is unusual in having good as well as troublesome side effects and the advantages of the method nearly always outweigh the disadvantages.

In those instances when oral contraceptives are contra-indicated or should be used with caution, surgical sterilization of one partner is very often an acceptable alternative.

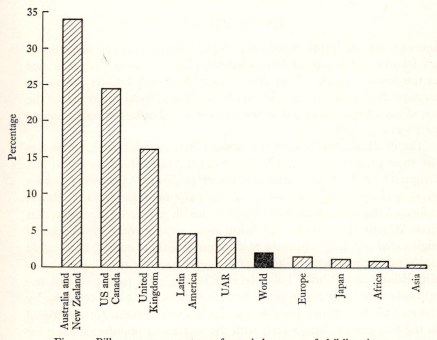

Fig. 25. Pill users as percentage of married women of childbearing age (15–44), 1968.

10 THE INTRAUTERINE DEVICE

HISTORICAL

Intrauterine and intracervical contraceptive devices, like all contemporary forms of birth control, have a lengthy history. Casanova's[1] reference to the use of a gold ball in this connection is well known and Guttmacher[2] has unearthed the inevitable anthropological reference to the use of such appliances (in this case a heat-treated rubber spiral) amongst preliterate peoples.

The medical forerunner of the modern intrauterine contraceptive was the stem pessary, first described and illustrated in the *Lancet* in 1868. Originally used for retroversions of the uterus, its contraceptive function must quickly have been noted, for ten years later Dr C. H. F. Routh informed the Obstetrical Section of the British Medical Association that these intrauterine stems were being worn permanently by women of high social standing to prevent conception. Routh, of course, thoroughly deplored the practice and accused his colleagues of 'teaching a way to sin without detection'. This piece of intelligence may have had the opposite consequences to those intended by the speaker; certainly by the end of the century intrauterine devices were prominently featured in the surgical catalogues and, with the increasing popular demand for birth control during the early years of this century, a wide range of alternative models was elaborated.

The most popular of these were the gold or gold-plated 'wishbone' and 'collar-stud' pessaries which were widely used by doctors in this country and in Germany. A disadvantage of both, however, was that the stem provided a vehicle for the infection of the uterus. It was through the accidental fracture of a 'collar-stud' pessary, resulting in the terminal ring being retained within the uterus, that the contraceptive efficacy of a completely intrauterine body was discovered.

The earliest form of strictly intrauterine contraceptive, a coil of silkworm thread secured by silver wire, was quickly superseded by an 18 mm diameter pliable ring of coiled silver wire. Such rings obviated the risk of infection and were popularized during the 1920s by Grafen-berg in Germany and by Norman Haire in Britain. The rings were inserted, usually without anaesthesia, by dilation of the cervix and the patient was re-examined annually. Although Grafenberg[3] claimed a high success rate for his ring the device became the subject of a great deal of controversy. Its insertion was accompanied by a high incidence of side effects which included pelvic inflammation, endometritis, septi-caemia and peritonitis; at least one recorded death was attributed to its use. Doctors were frequently harassed by applications from women, already pregnant, who expected in the course of fitting to obtain an abortion. The ring also suffered from the bad publicity which attended the use of the 'wishbone' pessary; despite the known and obvious dangers of this latter device it was still used extensively until fairly recently.

The most fundamental objection, however, to the Grafenberg ring lay in the undesirability of placing what was believed to be a chemically active foreign body within the uterus. For although the precise mode of action of the device was unknown, it was generally assumed that its effectiveness resulted from ionization of the metal with a consequent increase in the pH value of the uterus. After the mid-1930s the use of the Grafenberg ring was discountenanced by most doctors. A standard textbook on contraception, first published in 1938, classifies the Grafen-berg ring amongst 'harmful' methods and even in its latest edition,[4] in 1960, states: 'The use of intrauterine devices for birth control purposes is advisable only when other methods have failed repeatedly or are totally unacceptable'.

Although, in Western medical practice, the Grafenberg ring had fallen into disuse by the end of the Second World War, elsewhere it continued to be used on an experimental basis. In Japan, medical misgivings on the policy of birth control by legalized abortion stimulated an upsurge of contraceptive research in the 1950s. In the process a number of doctors undertook a re-examination of the intrauterine device and two of them, Kondo[5] and Ishihama,[6] achieved considerable success using rings constructed, predictably perhaps, from nylon and polythene. Their results were published in the Japanese medical press and attracted the attention of the American Population Council which, by the late 1950s, was looking around for promising avenues of research relevant to popu-lation control in underdeveloped countries.

Ishihama's work was immediately taken up in the US by clinicians who have now given their names to individual devices and whose work was financed by the Population Council. Between 1959 and 1962 the Council spent one and a half million dollars in support of this work. The outcome has been a collection of devices of various shapes and designs, made from polythene, together with a modified Grafenberg ring constructed from inert stainless steel.

MODE OF ACTION

Intrauterine contraceptive devices are an effective method of contraception (table 9) and, like oral contraceptives, they may act at more than one point in the reproductive cycle. No convincing explanation of their mode of action has been produced, although much has been discovered about ways in which they do not work. When the action of IUDs is understood it may be expected that there will be improvement in design and a rationalization of clinical advice concerning the method. Until that time animal experimentation and clinical follow-up have an important role to play in assessing the side effects and possible dangers of IUDs.

Ovulation, as determined by hormone output or endometrial biopsy, continues in the presence of an IUD. Living eggs, sperm and even fertilized eggs have been flushed from the Fallopian tubes of women having a salpingectomy or hysterectomy after some months of using a device.[7] The possibility of an IUD producing endocrine effects has been investigated and some interesting results have been obtained although none provides clear-cut evidence of the mode of action. Animals with intrauterine devices sometimes show a reduction in the number of corpora lutea and a shortening of the oestrus cycle has been reported in cows when the uterus is stretched. Changes in the output of FSH and LH have been demonstrated in women with IUDs but the work needs repeating on larger series. Some biopsy studies in women suggest that the maturation of the uterine epithelium may be delayed in the presence of an IUD. But the evidence is weak and the difficulty of dating the menstrual cycle, because of the excess bleeding that often occurs with a device, increases the uncertainty.

It has been suggested that an IUD might affect the motility of the reproductive tract. In a small group of superovulated monkeys Mastroianni was unable to recover eggs by tubal flushing when a device was in place, except when the tubes were ligated.[8] Large-scale follow-up of women with IUDs shows that although ectopic pregnancies still occur their incidence is less than expected. Among 22,400 women followed over

TABLE 9. *Clinical experience with IUDs*

Device	Number cycles studied	Pregnancies/ HWY*	Expulsions† (%)	Removals† (%)
Antigon	2,000	3·1	10·0	1·2
Birnberg bow (small)	21,111	11·3	4·5	18·1
(large)	33,221	5·3	2·4	16·5
DANA	33,373	3·9	4·5	3·1
Goldenstein ring	1,840	5·8	2·6	16·6
Hall-Stone ring	31,447	6·9	17·3	12·1
Lippes loop (A 22·5 mm)	19,935	4·9	23·9	18·2
(B 27·5 mm)	4,450	3·8	18·6	15·9
(C 30 mm)	29,334	2·5	21·9	13·6
(D 30 mm)	105,186	2·8	13·5	17·1
Margulies spiral (small)	6,966	3·4	38·7	23·6
(large)	36,146	1·6	25·2	26·6
Saf-T-coil	694	1·7	3·5	12·1
Silent protection (two types)	10,000	0–6	0–11	10
Szontagh device	18,791	11·6	7·5	20·5

* 1st year pregnancies only.   † Cumulative rate over 12 months.

300,000 cycles Tietze records only 26 ectopic pregnancies against the 200 to 300 which are predictable in a normal population of this size[9] and at first sight this appears to support the hypothesis that the device works by increasing tubal motility. However, serious doubt has been thrown on the original monkey experiments and Kelly and Marston have been unable to replicate these findings when ovulation was allowed to occur spontaneously.[10] The induction of ovulation with exogenous hormones, rather than the IUD, appears to have caused the increased uterine motility.

If ovulation and fertilization can occur with a device in situ and tubal transport is normal then the antifertility effect of IUDs is probably exerted later in development. In the presence of a foreign body the uterine environment may be hostile to the cleaving egg or there may be an interruption in the complex chain of events which takes place when the blastocyst attaches to the uterine wall. For instance, a device causes a migration of white cells into the uterine lumen.

The early stages of mammalian development are somewhat similar in man and the laboratory rodents: the blastocyst is small, invasive and the rate of development and size are comparable. The rodents differ from man in having a bicornuate uterus and multiple pregnancies making them convenient for experiments with intrauterine devices. A foreign body can be placed in one horn, where it will usually inhibit pregnancy while the other horn can be used as a control and will sustain normal development. Several workers have shown that if a thread is present in one horn of a rat's uterus at the time of mating but is removed before the beginning of implantation then development will proceed normally, but if it is left in place for more than the first three or four days of pregnancy then the experimental horn becomes infertile.[11] The device need not extend the full length of the uterine horn in order to exert a contraceptive effect. A short thread placed at the tubal end of the uterus will inhibit implantation throughout the experimental horn but a similar length of thread placed near the cervix will only prevent implantation in the areas of the uterus associated with the thread.

LONG TERM EFFECTS

In the absence of a thorough understanding of the function of IUDs it is still possible to comment on their side effects and possible long-term actions. Kar and his co-workers in India found that when a thread is placed in a rat uterus before puberty its contraceptive action continues for as long as it remains in place, but pregnancy recurs in the treated horn even if the device is removed after remaining in situ for a significant proportion of the reproductive life of the animal.[12] However, prolonged presence of the suture is associated with keratinized metaplasia in some animals and histological changes have been known to take place in the endometrium of rabbits since the work of Carlton and Phelps in 1933.[13] The possibility of malignant change must be faced although the available evidence does not give cause for alarm. Gross pathological changes of the type found in some animal experiments have not been found in man and one reason could be the lack of sterile precautions in many animal experiments. Both at the light and electron microscope level the response of the human endometrium to the presence of an IUD is mild.[14] The uterus may be particularly protected against severe long-term changes by the fact that the epithelium is only in contact with the device for not more than twenty days and then is cast off at the time of menstruation.

DEVICES

A satisfactory intrauterine device must be easy to insert, must remain in place and be associated with a low pregnancy rate and it must be easy to remove. Metal devices are the least flexible and may require cervical dilation under a general anaesthetic before insertion is possible. Some of the early plastic devices also suffered from this disadvantage but the polyethylene, nylon and silkworm gut devices that are in common use today are designed primarily for insertion without an anaesthetic.

The variety of devices available (figure 26) suggests that any uterine foreign body whatever its shape will have a contraceptive action. The simplest devices are the flexible, open-ended loops and coils usually made of plastic, although a stainless steel 'M'-shaped device is now available. They are easy to insert, have been widely used and have become the most popular choice among doctors. Closed rings and bows are more difficult to insert and carry a greater risk of perforation than the open devices but they have the advantage of a lower expulsion rate. Once the moulds have been made plastic devices can be produced very cheaply, although the commercial price may have little relation to the cost of manufacture. Cheap, simple, do-it-yourself devices which do not require industrialized manufacturing processes have also been devised. Grafenberg experimented with rings of silkworm gut, and hand-made rings of nylon thread have been shown to make acceptable devices by Zipper in Chile and Ragab in Egypt. Szontagh, in Hungary, has developed a simple closed device made by hand from 14 to 15 cm of nylon fishing line 0·7 mm thick welded into a loop on a flame.[15]

It is difficult to determine the normal shape and dimensions of the uterine cavity because most methods of investigation distort the lumen. In addition, the living uterus is a muscular organ undergoing contraction and relaxation. Attempts have been made to try to correlate uterine size with the design of IUDs and certain bows have been found to alter the cervical portion of the uterine cavity. X-ray studies suggest that many devices assume asymmetrical positions after insertion and may be distorted as the result of uterine contractions.

Nearly every device can be designed with or without a cervical 'tail'. The rigid plastic stem of the early Margulies' spirals has been abandoned because it was a potential tract for ascending infections and because it was difficult to prevent it impaling the male during intercourse. Fine nylon threads are attached to many devices and there is

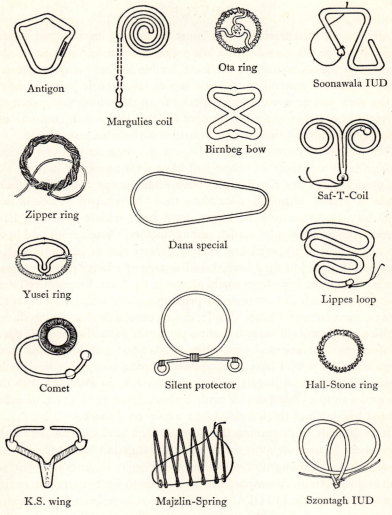

Antigon

Margulies coil

Ota ring

Soonawala IUD

Birnbeg bow

Saf-T-Coil

Zipper ring

Dana special

Yusei ring

Lippes loop

Comet

Silent protector

Hall-Stone ring

K.S. wing

Majzlin-Spring

Szontagh IUD

Fig. 26. Types of intrauterine device.

no evidence that they provide a route for infection. They are useful for checking that the device is in situ and for removing a device.

An introducer is necessary to pass an IUD through the cervical canal into the uterine cavity. For most closed rings and bows an introducer designed for the particular device is needed, but for open-ended loops and coils introducers are often interchangeable. Any introducer must be easily sterilized: it is best if the portion entering the cervical canal is pliable and there should be a stop which comes into contact with the external os and prevents the introducer passing too far into the uterine cavity (the risk of uterine perforation is greatest at the time of insertion). The Antigon is unusual among IUDs in that the tip of the collapsed device is the instrument for penetrating the cervix and the introducer remains at the external os. The pliable Zipper rings and Szontagh devices can be inserted with a metal hook or by a simple tube and plunger introducer.

STORAGE AND STERILIZATION

An IUD must be placed in the uterus under sterile conditions. While metal devices and introducers can be sterilized by boiling for five minutes, plastic introducers have a short life if boiled and no plastic device can be sterilized by heat—the polyethylene devices, for example, soften at 205 °F. However, nylon and polyethylene devices can be stored in an antiseptic solution. Benzalkonium chloride (Roccal, 1:750) is widely used and devices can remain indefinitely in screw-topped glass jars containing the solution. Unfortunately the action of the solution is slow, so that devices and introducers must be stored for a minimum of 24 hours in benzalkonium chloride prior to use.

As an alternative to benzalkonium chloride iodine may be used. It is an effective bactericidal and viricidal agent in concentrations of 1:100–1:5,000 (12 ml tincture of iodine to 100 ml water). Non-toxic, it will not give rise to irritation in any dilution below 1:500, and it will sterilize devices and introducers in one minute. Cheap, readily available and quick in action, it has much to recommend it to the physician who deals with small groups of patients or works outside his own surgery or hospital.

Certain devices are now provided with disposable introducers and supplied in sealed packs sterilized by gamma irradiation. They are more expensive than devices supplied loose but are convenient, especially when the operator is dealing with small series of cases at any one session.

INTERVIEW

The doctor must be prepared to devote as much or more time to explaining the method to the patient and answering her questions, as is spent inserting the device. If the doctor inserting the device does not have the overall care of the woman it is as well to ask why she has chosen this method of family planning. An unwillingness to use other methods of contraception may be a very good reason for having a device, but belief that it is less trouble than anything else is not always a valid argument.

A brief obstetric and medical history should be taken. It is difficult or impossible to pass an IUD through a nulliparous cervix without giving the patient a general anaesthetic. Women who have only had abortions or caesarian sections present a similar problem. An experienced operator may succeed in certain cases but more than usual caution is required, as a scar may predispose to perforation.

The risk of infection must be considered carefully in any woman who has not yet had a live child. If there is a history of current uterine infection or salpingitis an IUD should not be used and some reserve is necessary in the presence of past history of pelvic infection. Unfortunately, pelvic infection is often the consequence of illegal abortion and a choice may be necessary between the risks of exacerbating a possible intrauterine infection and the dangers inherent in another unwanted pregnancy.

A history of menorrhagia is not a contra-indication, although it is best treated before insertion and there should be good reasons why oral contraception cannot be used as a more suitable method of family planning. A haemoglobin estimate should be made if the woman is thought to be anaemic.

The woman should be shown the device and its position in the uterus should be explained, preferably with the aid of a model or diagram. For many women it is reassuring to be reminded that the Fallopian tubes leading into the uterus are very tiny and there is no possibility of the device 'getting lost inside'. In some women all knowledge of their body stops at the labia and it may not be out of place to emphasize that the device goes inside the uterus and not in the 'front passage'. A doctor may easily find certain women coming back pregnant having expelled the device and returned it to their vagina with a sincere conviction that it would be effective. The husband may be interested in what the method involves and sometimes it is useful to interview the couple together. The written permission of husband and wife should be available before inserting a device (see chapter 14).

The likelihood of heavy periods following insertion must be pointed out. A fair warning is the first step in dealing with the menorrhagia which may complicate the use of an IUD. It should be noted that some bleeding may follow insertion and the next period may begin some days early and be prolonged and heavy. At the same time encouragement may be given by telling the woman that in most cases the loss diminishes over the first few months of use. Vaginal tampons can be used when an IUD is in place.

It is important to state that IUDs have a failure rate. For most women exact figures or the personal experience of the doctor inserting the device may be useful. In other cases it may be simpler to couple a remark about failure rates with the comment that nothing in life is absolutely foolproof. One of the virtues of the IUD is that it can be used in patients who cannot manage with any other type of contra- ception and it can be of great benefit to women in the problem family group. However, in this group it is perhaps more than usually necessary to point out any side effects or drawbacks of the method. The real test of a contraceptive method is often what is said about it over the yard wall or in the supermarket and a failure that is known to be possible is more acceptable than one which was entirely unexpected.

The risk of spontaneous expulsion should be explained and women encouraged to return to the clinic or doctor if they think the device is being expelled. Most patients can be taught to feel the threads that protrude through the cervix when a 'tailed' device is used and this is particularly easy if the woman has used a diaphragm in the past. It is usually sufficient to check after each period. However, some women dislike feeling their cervix or are unnecessarily worried by the procedure. (In such cases the husband may become a competent guardian of his wife's intrauterine contraceptive.) There is a small magnet embedded in the Antigon and its presence can be checked by a magnetometer.

It is important to remember that sexual customs vary among different social, religious and ethnic groups. Some men appear to be aware of the presence of cervical threads and one member of a couple, by accident or design, may pull on the threads and remove the device. This is a disadvantage in couples where attitudes to family planning vary from day to day and may account for the high 'expulsion' rate in some social groups. Among the Irish, on the other hand, there are taboos against digital exploration of the vagina. For certain religious groups menstru- ation is a time of uncleanness. Moslem women are forbidden to pray or have intercourse during a period and orthodox Jews are forbidden to have intercourse for seven days after the menstruation ceases.[16] For these groups the prolonged loss that is commonly associated with an IUD can be more than usually tiresome, especially if they fail to distinguish between true menstrual loss and slight intermenstrual bleeding.

INSERTION

It is possible to insert IUDs single handed, but an assistant is of great value, especially when a number of women are being fitted at one session and when other than γ-ray sterilized devices are being used. When IUDs are inserted in large numbers occasions will arise when the aid of specialist services will be needed. X-rays may be required to locate a device, a general anaesthetic may be needed if a device proves difficult to remove and there is a risk of perforation or pelvic infection requiring hospital care. Intrauterine devices are best inserted by doctors having, if possible, some gynaecological experience. However, nurses and mid-wives can be trained to insert devices under medical supervision and if a choice has to be made between not having an IUD service for a community and one involving para-medical staff the latter is preferable.

A device can be inserted at any time in the menstrual cycle, but there are several advantages in choosing a time at or near a period. Menstruation excludes the possibility of an early pregnancy, instrumentation of the cervix is easiest at this time and the small amount of traumatic bleeding which follows insertion is not noticed. Unfortunately, it is difficult to arrange for women to attend a busy clinic at a particular phase of their cycle. Insertion is exceptionally easy to carry out at the time of delivery, or in the first day or two of the puerperum. When performed at this time there is an increased risk of expulsion (8 to 34 per cent) but the perforation and infection rates are not raised. Insertion in the weeks immediately following delivery carries a higher-than-normal risk of perforation, migration through the uterine wall after insertion and an increased chance of expulsion (8 per cent) and it is therefore contra-indicated. Insertion at eight weeks post partum has a normal expulsion rate.[17] In practice, an IUD can be considered at the post-natal visit and either fitted immediately or within a week or two. Insertion at delivery is worth offering to the woman who has chosen this method when discussing future family planning earlier in the pregnancy. Insertion has been performed at the time of legal abortion. No increased risk of infection, perforation or expulsion was found.[18] The

method is particularly valuable because most women are strongly motivated towards family planning at the time of a termination.

The equipment which it is advisable to have when inserting IUDs is
detailed in Appendix IV. A bimanual pelvic examination and speculum
examination are made noting any evidence of pelvic infection (such as
tenderness in the fornices or pain on moving the cervix), the presence
of fibroids and the position and type of uterus. Intramural or subserosal
fibroids do not affect an IUD but submucosal fibroids, distorting the
uterine lumen, are a contra-indication. Endocervicitis is relatively
common and if severe it is best treated by cautery before inserting an
IUD. There is no evidence that passing instruments past a mild cervical
infection is followed by an increased risk of intrauterine infection.

A firm couch at a convenient height for the operator, a good speculum
and a bright light are essential. Either a bivalve or a Cusko speculum
are best. Freshly sterilized instruments must be available for each
patient and it is convenient to be able to transfer them from the sterilizer
onto a clean trolley or large tray.

Insertion is most easily performed with the patient in lithotomy position. The hands are scrubbed, sterile gloves should be used (disposable
γ-ray sterilized gloves are useful) but a mask need not be worn. A
speculum is passed and the cervix clearly illuminated. It can be useful
to hold the cervix with a tenanculum and the more inexperienced the
operator the more this may be necessary. Other situations in which it
is useful to stabilize the cervix are those in which the uterus is retroverted, when the cervix is relatively inaccessible, if the uterus is poorly
supported and very mobile or if any difficulty is found passing sound
or inserting the introducer.

A uterine sound is passed in order to discover the direction and tone
of the cervical canal. In addition, the position of the uterus as determined by the pelvic examination will be confirmed and the size of the
uterine cavity can be estimated. There is a great deal of variation in the
anatomy of the cervical canal. The canal may not be centrally placed in
the external os or there may be blind passages and sometimes the sound
must be partially withdrawn and reinserted before it will enter the
uterine cavity. It should be possible to pass the sound with the minimum
of force letting it rest between the finger and thumb of the right hand
like a loosely held pencil. If the sound can be passed into the uterus,
but some tightness of the cervical canal is found then it is useful to pass
a dilator to the same size as the introducer (Hega 2). This reduces the

possibility of bleeding when the rim of the introducer is passed up the cervical canal.

Plastic devices must be left in the introducer for the shortest possible interval or they will fail to return to their original shape after insertion. Some devices are picked up by their own tails and pulled into the introducer, and others are inserted into the introducer by manipulation through the transparent sterile packet in which it is supplied. The Lippes' loop must be fed into the proximal end of the introducer and then pushed along the introducer until the tip (opposite the threads) almost protrudes from the distal end. A no-touch sterile technique is advisable when handling devices. A small amount of chlortetracycline paste on the tip of the introducer is used by some operators.

When the introducer has been passed along the cervical canal it is important to rotate it so that the device is expelled in the transverse plane of the uterus and not in the sagittal plane where it will distort the lumen giving rise to pain. A device should be inserted slowly over an interval of 5 to 15 seconds and the patient's face, rather than her perineum should be observed during insertion to watch for any signs of discomfort or shock. In the case of the Lippes' loop the plunger should be withdrawn before removing the introducer or the threads may become caught and the device pulled out again. The threads should be trimmed to about 2 to 3 cm of the external os. The most common error when introducing a device is not to pass the introducer past the internal cervical os. The end of the device is then left in the cervical canal which gives rise to pain and predisposes to expulsion.

It is possible to insert IUDs without any discomfort to the patient but dilation and handling the cervix may cause pain and shock. If pain occurs the patient should be asked if she wishes the procedure to continue or if she would rather return for another attempt. If there has been considerable manipulation of the cervix before insertion is attempted it may be best to postpone the operation until another occasion when the patient will be more familiar with the procedure and the operator with her cervix. Shock is more serious and need not be related to the degree of pain. The patient may become unconscious, the skin blanched and clammy, the pulse slow, thready and perhaps unobtainable. However, this rarely happens without warning and often the patient will have complained of feeling faint, and commonly there will have been something difficult or unusual about the insertion such as repeated attempts to find the cervical canal. The woman always recovers after a short interval. The operator usually removes the device to relieve his own distress but there is no evidence that this is necessary if the device is correctly placed in the uterine cavity.

FOLLOW-UP VISITS

The patient should be seen some time in the next menstrual cycle, she should be asked about her last period, which she will probably say was heavier than usual, but she may be reassured that the next one will probably be more normal. Occasional massive flooding will be reported, perhaps with clots, and the woman may have had to take to her bed. It may be necessary to remove the device immediately, but more commonly either the woman or the doctor will have reasons why she should persevere for at least one more cycle. Oral iron should be prescribed and another appointment made for the following month. The timing of subsequent follow-up visits is determined by the patient's age, whether she considers her family complete, her intelligence and the resources of the doctor or clinic. Most women can be left for a year after the first check visit and some for considerably longer. But the young girl who may have had one or more babies adopted but still looks forward to marriage and a family of her own may need seeing every six months or less. An experienced nurse under the guidance of a doctor can do some follow-up examinations. In the context of a domiciliary family planning service check visits can be done at home.

It is important to make a real effort never to lose contact with women using IUDs—although the task can be a great burden. In particular, no survey of IUDs has yet run long enough to indicate if it is in a woman's best interest to leave a device in situ until the end of her reproductive life or renew it at intervals. The WHO Scientific Group on intrauterine devices concluded that on the bases of present evidence an IUD could remain in place until the menopause.[19] From the general point of view the risks involved in any method of contraception cannot be fully assessed until a statistically significant group of women has been followed for a generation.

SIDE EFFECTS

1   Death

A questionnaire circulated on behalf of the American Food and Drug Administration to over 8,000 Fellows of the American College of Obstetricians and Gynecologists elicited reports of ten deaths associated with

IUDs. In four cases death was due to inflammatory disease within one month of insertion, in another four cases death occurred between six weeks and two years after insertion and may have been connected with the device and in the remaining two cases the association was thought to be coincidental. Over 500 cases of severe illness were reported: 350 due to infection and the remainder to perforation.

It is difficult to estimate how many IUDs have been inserted in America or how many women-years of use are involved in the above reports, but it is probably in the region of one to two million.

2 Bleeding

The mean blood loss at menstruation is about 45 ml and the loss is highest in women nearing the menopause. A loss of 60 to 80 ml is associated with a low haemoglobin and must be considered pathological.[20] Menorrhagia is the most common and troublesome side effect of an intrauterine device and gives rise to a measurable anaemia in about half the women fitted.[21] For the first few months after insertion most patients report an increase in the duration and amount of their menstrual loss. It is common for the periods to begin one or two days earlier than usual, with a light loss and then for the main, heavier loss to be recognized. Clots may be passed, there may be some pain and the heavy loss may continue for four or five days or more. It may then cease or trail off with irregular spotting which in some cases continues until the next period. On the whole the first two or three cycles after insertion are the worst, but even initially severe bleeding can settle to tolerable levels with time.

So far no valid trials have been carried out on the rational treatment of IUD menorrhagia. There is an impression that bleeding is less when a device is inserted six to eight weeks after childbirth or when insertion is covered for one or two cycles by oral contraceptives in women changing from the Pill to the coil. Vitamin C has been used on the theory that it might protect against capillary fragility. But at present the most rational treatment of heavy bleeding associated with an IUD is reassurance, careful observation, taking measures to avoid anaemia (oral iron, of a type the woman can tolerate, should be used freely) and removal when necessary.

3 Pain

Uterine cramp at the time of insertion is common and there may be some dysmenorrhea if the device provokes a heavy flow, but pain at other times in the cycle is unusual. Analgesics, like codeine, can be prescribed. Pain is the primary complaint leading to removal in 2 to 3 per cent of patients.[22] Sometimes pain is associated with an anxious personality or with religious beliefs that do not accept contraception freely.

4 Expulsion

Depending upon the type of device used, between 4 and 30 per cent are expelled in the first year after insertion. Expulsion is particularly common at the time of menstruation and most common of all at the first post-insertion period. High parity protects against expulsion.[9] Many women are aware of 'cramp' at the time of expulsion or 'feel it coming out'; others discover the device on the sanitary towel or in the vagina.

The purpose of a cervical tail is to allow the patient or doctor to check that the device is in place. If the threads cannot be palpated either the device has been expelled or has been rotated by myometrical contractions drawing the threads inside the cervix. Often a device can be detected by probing with a uterine sound. (Instrumental probes that can distinguish between metal, plastic and tissue have been invented.)[23] Nearly all devices are radio opaque but the X-ray location of a device must be carried out with caution in case the device has been expelled and the woman is already pregnant. It is not always easy from an X-ray examination to exclude the possibility that a device has perforated the uterus.

When an open-ended device is expelled it is usually worth re-inserting another device of the same type. If expulsion is repeated then a closed bow should be considered. The expulsion rates for large bows is $4 \cdot 5 \pm 0 \cdot 5$ per 100 women over the first year.

5 Infection

The vagina, like the skin, has its own bacterial flora and the cervical canal is infected in up to 80 per cent of normal women. Cervical infection is not relieved by swabbing with antiseptic solutions. The uterine cavity is probably sterile unless there is some predisposing factor to infection such as cervical cancer.[24] It is difficult to obtain material for culture and the only reliable method is by a transfundal approach at laparotomy. When this method is used in the case of the IUDs, infection is always found immediately following insertion but the uterus appears to become sterile again during the next cycle.[25] It must be concluded that it is impossible to avoid carrying infection from the cervical canal into the uterine cavity at the time of insertion, but in nearly every case the uterus is able to deal with this infection.

However, in rare cases clinically significant uterine infection does complicate insertion. In many of these there is a previous history of pelvic infection. The diagnosis can be difficult as pain may also be a sign of uterine distension. If there is uterine pain, tenderness on examination and a suspicious cervical discharge, a smear should be taken for culture and in nearly all cases the device should be removed.

Pyrexia is a serious sign, the device must be removed, and antibiotics commenced as soon as a smear has been taken.

Pelvic infection is suspected more often than it is proved in women using IUDs. Lippes[22] found 23 cases of suspected pelvic infection in 1,673 patients fitted with loops but in 14 cases the diagnosis was not substantiated. Tietze reports a 2 per cent infection rate per year.[26] The possibility of an ectopic gestation must be remembered as part of the differential diagnosis of a woman with abdominal pain, uterine tenderness and an IUD.

In theory it is possible to transfer infectious hepatitis between patients when non-disposable introducers are used, as insertion is always associated with some bleeding from the cervical canal, but no cases have been reported.

TABLE 10. *Uterine perforations with IUDs*

Device	Uterine perforations/1,000 insertions
Lippes loop	0·4
Margulies spiral	0·3
Hall-Stone ring	1·0
Birnberg bow	5·0–8·0

6 Perforation

The incidence of perforation varies with the type of device and is highest in the first six weeks post partum (tables 10 and 11). Perforation is most likely at insertion but a device may migrate through the uterine wall some time later. Perforation is often symptomless and in the case of an open-ended device laparotomy is rarely justified. However, intestinal obstruction has been recorded after Birnberg bows have perforated[26] and surgical removal should be considered in these cases.

TABLE 11. *Uterine perforations for post partum insertion of bows*

Weeks post partum	Uterine perforations/1,000 insertions
2–5	34·0
6	31·0
7–12	14·0–4·0
13+	2·0

7 Pregnancy

Pregnancy can occur if the device is lost silently, if it is expelled and replaced in the vagina by the woman and it can occur when it is correctly positioned. Not all authors distinguish between these categories. Some women who become pregnant may be lost to follow-up because they accept the pregnancy or because they have an illegal abortion and some series (table 9) may underestimate the failure rate.

The risk of failure with the device in situ appears to be directly related to the mass of the plastic in the device. The failure rate is higher in small loops than in large ones and higher still for Birnberg bows and the Szontagh device.

Human implantation is interstitial, the fetal membranes expanding in the thickness of the endometrium. The uterine lumen is obliterated and a device, if present, is caught between the decidual capsularis and decidua parietalis. Therefore the device remains outside the fetal membranes; it is related to maternal tissues and not to the embryo. The surmise that a retained IUD will not be teratogenic is supported by those follow-up studies which have been carried out.[26] It may be that certain types of pathological pregnancy such as retained placenta or placenta praevia, will tend to escape the contraceptive action of the device (as is the case in tubal pregnancies). Such abnormalities would then appear to be spuriously common and the reports which have been published need to be analysed as part of a very large series of cases. Pregnancies with the device in situ have a higher spontaneous abortion rate than pregnancies which occur after a device has been expelled, but the difference is very slight[26] and may be confused by criminal abortions.

PLANNED PREGNANCIES

Following removal of a device one in every three women becomes pregnant in the next succeeding cycle, three-quarters within six months and nine out of ten within one year, which are perfectly normal rates for the population.[26]

EVALUATION

Intrauterine contraceptives have the unique advantage that once inserted they require no further action by the patient. In addition, they have a lower failure rate than any other method except the Pill, they do not interfere with lactation, and they are inexpensive to produce. Allowing for removals and expulsions the method appears to be suitable for three out of four women (figure 27). Intrauterine devices are a valuable addition to the available methods of contraception and can prove successful in women of any age, and of all degrees of initiative and intelligence.

There are three groups of women for whom they appear to be especially suited. (1) For those who dislike the cap and cannot or will not take oral contraceptives they are often the only possible method. (2) Among women who have completed their families and require simple and effective family planning until the menopause they are worth serious consideration. (3) They are the method of choice among parous women who forget or become muddled on oral contraceptives or whose way of life is such that they are unlikely to use consistently any patient-dependent method of contraception. For this reason IUDs are commonly used by domiciliary family planning services.

For some the IUD will prove the answer to the parous woman's prayer; for others it will give rise to a tiresome series of side effects. The reputation of the method will to some extent depend on the way in which the after care of the patient is carried out. For the majority of women there must be a considerable readiness to remove the device if trouble begins to be apparent. For the minority who make up the problem family group reluctance to remove the device may prove to be in the best long-term interest of the patient.

The choice of device is determined partly by familiarity and availability. The large loops have a low failure rate and an acceptable expulsion rate. The bows have a higher perforation rate and failure rate but are expelled less often. Some devices such as the Szontagh IUD appear to have high failure rates but give rise to less bleeding than others and may prove particularly valuable for multiparous women who are gravely anaemic at the time a device is inserted.

In many cases it is probable that IUDs are used to curtail reproduction when a woman has achieved a desired number of children (or a

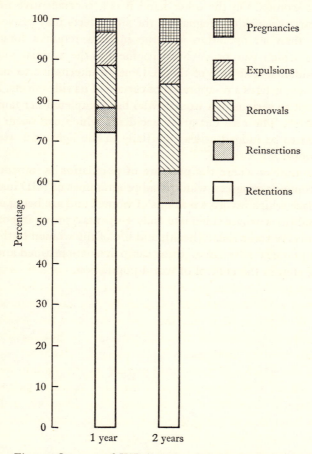

Fig. 27. Outcome of IUD insertions based on 1,798 cases using Lippes loop C (5·4 per cent lost to follow-up).

number in excess of the desired number), rather than as a method of postponing a family early in marriage or for spacing births within a family. They tend to be fitted to women in the latter half of their reproductive life and it is uncommon for a doctor to be asked to remove a device in order that the woman can initiate a further pregnancy. Thus, in many cases, the IUD is being used as an alternative to tubal ligation. It has the advantages of being reversible, of not involving the risks of an anaesthetic or laparotomy and of not requiring hospitalization and time away from the family—a fact of some importance among certain highly fertile women. On the other hand it is a contraceptive method which still carries a risk of pregnancy, the side effects may prove more troublesome than an operation and the method requires long-term medical care which can prove burdensome for the woman and her medical attendants. The role of the IUD as an alternative to surgical sterilization necessitates a re-appraisal of certain of its side effects. Pelvic infection is not so serious in a woman who has completed her family as in a bride of 18. The rare but grave accidents which can occur using an IUD need to be judged at least partially in the light of a woman's previous history.

In those countries where the pressure of population is impeding all social and economic progress, widespread programmes of IUD insertion are taking place which involves millions of women and are being undertaken in conditions where adequate follow-up may prove impossible. This must involve some risk to health and life of the women but, in the absence of a practical alternative, these campaigns are justified and may prove a vital step in the control of world population.

11 MINOR METHODS

As a hangover from birth control's historical and clandestine past there persist, even in contemporary societies and amongst otherwise sophisticated sections of the population, practices and techniques which range from the quaint to the grotesque. None of these can be particularly effective and a few may be positively dangerous; the doctor should be aware of their existence and, in view of the many safe, reliable and aesthetic alternatives available, feel justified in discouraging their use.

DOUCHING

The flushing of the vaginal tract immediately after intercourse was first recommended in Knowlton's *Fruits of Philosophy* and has always been more popular in the United States than in England. In both countries, however, it had considerable popularity in the early decades of this century and a variety of appliances, including wall-cans, bulb-syringes and whirling-sprays, were sold for the purpose. Douching solutions were usually prepared from household substances such as vinegar, alum, salt or soap.[1] In developing countries Coca Cola is very popular as a vaginal douche, its low pH making it a not unsuitable choice.

Studies in the United States have revealed that up to 28 per cent of women married between 1935 and 1955 had used this method at some time (though a third claimed to have used it 'for vaginal cleanliness only') compared with only 3 per cent in the English PIC survey in 1959. None of the newly married women interviewed in Hull in 1965 admitted to using the method and there is no doubt that it will disappear as the married population becomes more sophisticated in its contraceptive choices. A major disadvantage of this method, apart from its doubtful efficacy, is that it interrupts the relaxation which normally follows intercourse; the apparatus required for efficient douching must also be an embarrassment in most households.

COITUS RESERVATUS

A technique which is closely related to coitus interruptus and which calls for an even greater degree of male constraint is known as coitus reservatus, male continence, magnetation or karezza. In this case there is no ejaculation either within or outside the vagina; instead the man avoids a too close approach to orgasm and allows detumescence to take place slowly over a prolonged period. Frequently mentioned in the erotic literature of most cultures it is best known as the prescribed practice of the Oneida Community, a voluntary colony, established by John Humphrey Noyes near New York in 1869, which was devoted to perfectionism in eugenic selection, sexual relations and the production of silver-plated tableware.

Noyes, like other writers on the subject, claimed as the main advantage of coitus reservatus that it allowed the satisfaction of complete, or even multiple, orgasm to the female partner. Male self-control was to be assisted by spiritual contemplation; as a secular alternative one of Kingsley Amis's heroes has more recently recommended the conjugation of Latin verbs. Except perhaps in old age, coitus reservatus would not appear to be a particularly appropriate method of birth control, though Marie Stopes suggested[2] that its use was more widespread than was usually imagined and that people who claimed that 'continence is the only right thing when children are not desired' were referring, not to abstinence, but to coitus reservatus. Because this practice, unlike coitus interruptus, involves no ejaculation, it is a method to which the Catholic Church takes no particular objection.[3]

COITUS SAXONICUS

This consists of normal unprotected coitus up to the point of ejaculation when the man exerts pressure on his perineum so as to cause the spermatozoa to be refluxed into the bladder. No external ejaculation takes place and the ejaculate is later emitted during urination. This appears to be a contraceptive method suited only to blacksmiths, though the erotic literature recommends that the female partner should be trained to do the pressing. It is a practice which should be discouraged in all circumstances.

'HOLDING BACK'

It is a commonly held belief that female orgasm involves a discharge comparable to male ejaculation and on this erroneous notion has been erected the theory that by 'holding back' from orgasm a woman may avoid impregnation. The idea is completely mistaken; Kinsey revealed[3] that a large number of women never achieve orgasm, or do so only once or twice in their lives, but this does not prevent them becoming pregnant.

SPONGES AND TAMPONS

A form of female contraception which was popular until recently and which still has some adherents in the older age-groups consists of the use of a sponge in conjunction with either a spermicidal paste, olive oil or soap. This may be a partly effective method of birth control but there appears to be no reason why a woman who feels able to use such a method should not be persuaded to transfer to the more hygienic cap or diaphragm.

Even less satisfactory are pads of cotton or wool which have been used in the same way as the sponge as occlusive devices. Although perfectly permissible in an emergency, their prolonged use is to be severely discouraged.

GAMIC MALE APPLIANCES

Described by its manufacturers as 'a male internal contraceptive', this device consists of a short nylon stem with an attached latex sac which is folded into the hollow stem before use. The stem is then inserted in the urethra and, on ejaculation, the spermatozoa are forced into the sac which is extruded from its stem in the process. The dangers of infection and of urethral damage are obvious.

PROLONGED LACTATION

The belief that a woman cannot conceive whilst breast-feeding has a long-established place in the folklore of birth control although medical writers have traditionally rejected its validity. Recently, however, it has been conceded that the notion has some basis in fact, a suggestion which was first made[4] by a historical demographer on the basis of birth and death records in a Normandy village during the period 1674–1742. It was noted that the interval between successive births differed by an average of ten and a half months depending upon whether the older child survived or died during the first year of infancy. Because, in the former case, the death of the older infant invariably preceded the subsequent conception it was concluded that the death led to cessation of lactation which in turn gave rise to ovulation and conception.

In a review of the clinical data, which are slight, Tietze has suggested[5] that prolonged lactation has the effect of lengthening the normal period of post partum amenorrhea, which usually lasts for two and a half months in a non-lactating mother, to eleven or twelve months. He recognizes the possibility that lactation may delay pregnancy, even after resumption of ovulation, by interfering with the process of nidation through hormonal action on the uterus and recommends research on this neglected aspect of human reproduction. It is possible that the method is more effective among poorly nourished women, where lactation presents more of a strain, than among the exceptionally healthy women of the present-day Western world.

It seems possible then that lactation may provide some immunity against conception for approximately ten months, but this is a statement of a physiological fact rather than the basis for a programme of fertility control. Although the average couple, having a family of two or three children, will enjoy the bonus of a few months freedom from contraceptive use they would be well advised to return to positive birth control practice as soon as possible after the third delivery.

INTRASCROTAL HYPERTHERMIA

In all mammals (except the whale and the elephant) having a body temperature above 36 °C spermatogenesis takes place outside the abdomen. There are numerous examples of raised scrotal temperature leading to infertility. The anatomy of the testicular vessels is thought to act as a heat exchanger and a varicocele, which disrupts the normal function, may impair fertility. Merino sheep fail to breed in the hotter parts of Australia and amongst men in Maharashtra State in India who, by custom, wear tight scrotal suspenders 24 hours a day subfertility is common. Yet 30 per cent of one group who abandoned the suspender subsequently fathered children. Robinson and Rock have shown that a jockstrap, with disposable paper insulation, worn during working hours for several weeks, causes a 75 per cent reduction in sperm count.[6] Perhaps the idea deserves further investigation—especially in hot countries.

12 STERILIZATION

INTRODUCTION

There is a long, often bizarre, history of surgical attempts to control human fertility. Some methods were mutilating, cruelly painful and dangerous and hysterectomy and female castration have been practised in certain primitive societies.

The first surgical sterilization was carried out in America in 1897. Initially the operation was limited to eugenic considerations, such as severe mental defect. When the British Departmental Committee on Sterilization, under the chairmanship of Sir Lawrence Brock, reported in 1934 the scope of sterilization was envisaged as including the healthy who might transmit genetic disease. The need to change the law was considered as an 'act of social justice' but no legislation was enacted by the British Parliament and the subject was displaced from the forum of public debate by the Second World War.[1] In mainland Europe the gross and inhuman misuse of sterilization by Nazi doctors caused a reaction against sterilization which it has taken a generation to overcome.

Today, the use of sterilizing procedures is increasing in most countries. In a survey of 2,414 United States couples carried out by the Scripps Foundation for Research in Population Problems in 1964 it was found that among white American couples, where the wife was between 18 and 39, 10 per cent had had a sterilizing operation.[2] Six out of ten had vasectomies or tubal ligation and four had sterilizing operations in the course of gynaecological treatment. By 1956 in the United States the yearly rate of sterilization was 1 per cent.

In Britain and America tubal ligation is performed more commonly than vasectomy. About 20,000 tubal ligations are performed annually in Britain and the number is rising yearly. One or two far-sighted centres have a long history of using female sterilization as a valuable and integral part of the medical care of the community. Among social classes IV and V acceptance of the technique grows slowly and a consistent and per-

153

sistent policy is required. Baird[3] has described how, in Aberdeen, post partum tubal ligation was first offered in 1930 to women between 35 and 40 with eight or more children. Over the years the criteria were relaxed and by 1966 7·2 per cent of the women over 30 in the city had been sterilized and 12·6 per cent over 35 and among women of all ages over a quarter of those with five or more children were sterilized. In a hospital survey in a poor quarter of Hongkong post partum sterilization was performed on 13·6 per cent of admissions.[4]

Although interest in vasectomy has lagged behind that in tubal ligation a significant number of operations is now performed in both developed and developing countries. In the United States over 50,000 vasectomies take place yearly. In the United Kingdom 1,600 operations were done under the auspices of the Simon Population Trust between 1960–6. In India over $1\frac{1}{2}$ million vasectomies have been performed in the past decade and although the possibility of obtaining a transistor radio in return for being sterilized has captured the imagination of western onlookers, its impact on Indian peasants remains to be determined. The number of vasectomies in Pakistan has risen from 500 in 1965 to 21,000 in the first half of 1968. In Central and Eastern Europe the operation is almost unknown but national laws on the subject are being altered.

TECHNIQUES

It is imperative that the doctor should explain the nature and consequences of the operation to the patient. The less intelligent the patient and the more difficult communication, the greater the importance of the preliminary discussion and explanation, but the doctor must also avoid falling into the trap of assuming that all well-educated people are fully and accurately informed about their reproductive systems. The basic question every patient wants answered is 'Will I be the same, doctor?' 'Will I still be like a woman?' 'Will I behave like a man?' It is very common to equate sterilization with castration and even those who realize the two are different may need reassurance. The doctor can explain that the testes or ovaries are left behind and that they make the hormones responsible for sexual behaviour. Some kind of illustration or model may be helpful. Sometimes the most helpful thing is for a patient to meet someone who has been surgically sterilized. Men sometimes want to know what happens to the sperm that continue to be formed. They may also need to be told that the ejaculate comes mainly from the accessory glands and that they will notice no difference in amount. Women may be puzzled about the fate of the eggs.

The doctor should try to see the husband and wife together at a pre-operative interview. Legal aspects of sterilization are considered in chapter 14.

1 Male

The operation should be done when the patient can be away from work for a day or two—a weekend is sufficient.

A brief history should be taken and the site of the operation examined. Diabetes and haemophilia are immediately relevant to the operation and it is useful to ask specific questions concerning drug allergies, particularly to antibiotics or local anaesthetics. If a varicocele, hydrocele, hernia or a cyst of the reproductive tract is discovered the operative procedure may have to be redesigned.

It is easiest to ask the man to shave his own pubic hair, and if a general anaesthetic is to be used no food should be taken on the morning of the operation. Usually, the threat that a junior nurse will be detailed to shave the region is sufficient to ensure patient co-operation, but some men lack the self-discipline to abstain from food and most surgeons prefer to admit the patient to hospital for one night prior to the operation if a general anaesthetic is planned.

General anaesthesia allows a smaller incision to be made, more careful dissection of the vas deferens and better haemostasis. It also speeds the time the operation takes. It may be requested, insisted upon, or the surgeon may feel it is necessary for the more apprehensive of men. Local anaesthesia eliminates the very remote risks of inhalation anaesthetics, it permits the surgeon to act single handed and it cuts down the time the patient must spend in the clinic. Two per cent xylocaine with adrenaline (1 part in 200,000) is a suitable local anaesthetic. The adrenaline should be omitted if the patient has a history of heart disease. Two to 5 ml are usually sufficient at the site of the skin incision. A tranquillizer may be given one to two hours preoperatively. Before incising the skin the area should be washed with an aqueous antiseptic.

The vas deferens is about 2·5 mm in diameter, it has a characteristic cord-like feel when palpated between finger and thumb and it forms one component of the spermatic cord which also contains the testicular artery, arteries to the vas and cremaster muscle, the pampiniform plexus of veins, lymphatic vessels, the testicular nerves and genital branch of the genito-femoral nerve. At operation the vas must be separated from the other structures. Mistakes can occur and when possible the material that is removed should be sent for histology. Congenital anomalies are not uncommon in the reproductive tracts and reduplication of the vas deferens (mesonephric duct) has been described.

The vas deferens is approximately 45 cm (18 in) long. The part related to the posterior surface of the testes is highly convoluted but between the upper pole of the testes and the superficial inguinal ring it is readily accessible and the spermatic cord in this region can be palpated through the skin. Several incisions to expose the spermatic cord are possible. Bilateral vasectomy can be performed through a single midline incision made posteriorly in the scrotum. However, pulling the cord across may cause troublesome bleeding from small vessels. Probably the best technique is to palpate the cord through the skin at the point where the scrotum joins the body. It is useful to lift up the spermatic cord in a fold of skin and pass a syringe needle through the skin fold, posterior and well clear of the cord, anchoring it in place, although care must be taken to avoid damaging any veins. A short incision is then made over the cord.

A loop of spermatic cord is delivered through the skin incision and the vas deferens carefully and thoroughly separated from the remaining structures in the cord. The cremaster muscle should be incised longitudinally, not transversely. If local anaesthetic is used the patient will complain of pain unless the cord is handled with great gentleness and it is usually necessary to infiltrate the vas itself. Two small artery forceps are applied to the vas about 2 cm apart and the intervening portion cut away. Although it increases the effectiveness of the operation to remove a long length of vas deferens, if reamastomosis was ever to be attempted the operation would be more difficult. The cut ends can be either crushed and ligated with black silk (3/0) or cauterized with a needle electrode placed in the lumen. It is useful to draw the sheath of the vas over the distal stump. The vas deferens should be held with fine Allis forceps during these procedures because, if either end is dropped, the muscular coat will contract and it may be impossible to retrieve.

Good haemostasis is of more than usual importance. Bleeding may occur from the artery to the vas deferens and if possible this should be ligated. The skin incision is best closed with black silk sutures as this procedure will ensure that the patient returns to the doctor at least once. The sutures can be removed after three or four days. An analgesic tablet should be given after the operation. The intact vas deferens is a mechanical support to the testes and after vasectomy some men feel a dragging discomfort in the scrotum. In addition, there may be short-term swelling and testicular tenderness. Y-fronted underpants relieve much of the post-operative discomfort but sometimes a supporting bandage is required.

Most men resume sexual intercourse within four weeks of the operation and some within three days to a week. *A man is not sterile immediately after vasectomy* as mature sperm remain in the vas deferens and accessory glands proximal to the ligature. The patient should have his semen examined eight weeks after the operation and during this interval he should have intercourse with reasonable frequency but the couple must continue to use an adequate form of contraception. A masturbatory semen specimen should be collected into a glass container at body temperature and be examined for the presence of sperm within two hours of being collected. Some surgeons require two negative semen tests one month apart. Many men who have had a vasectomy (32 out of 73 in one series[5]) fail to keep all their follow-up appointments and failures sometimes occur for this reason. It might be possible to inject the vas deferens towards the prostate with a spermicidal liquid at operation, though the procedure is so far untried.

2 Female

(*a*) OPERATIONS ON THE FALLOPIAN TUBES

Tubal ligation, partial excision or total salpingectomy are the commonest and most acceptable sterilizing procedures in women.

Post partum sterilization and tubal ligation by the vaginal route can be performed under local anaesthesia, but supplementary inhalation anaesthesia is often needed and in the absence of special circumstances a general anaesthetic is indicated.

(*b*) ELECTIVE OPERATIONS

A medical and gynaecological history should be taken and a careful pelvic examination carried out. When a cervical smear is taken the result should be available before operation. Care should be taken to see that the woman is not pregnant and it should be remembered that, if tubal ligation is performed in the second half of the cycle, fertilization and tubal transport of the ovum may have already occurred and some surgeons routinely perform a dilatation and curettage when tying the tubes. Material should be sent for histology as cases of uterine disease may be diagnosed. In cases of prolapse, tubal ligation may be combined with a repair operation and on rare occasions there may be gynaecological indications for a hysterectomy rather than a sterilizing procedure on the tubes.

There is a great deal of variation in the technique used to occlude the Fallopian tubes, suggesting that while many different methods will work none is perfect. The simplest techniques are those of Pomeroy and Madlener. In the former, the middle third of the tube is grasped with dissecting forceps and the loop that is raised up is ligatured with fine catgut and excised. In Madlener's operation[6] a length of tube is crushed and held with a clamp for one minute, it is ligated with a non-absorbable suture and no tissue is removed. Both methods are rapid and there is little cause for haemorrhage but failures are commoner than with more complex methods.

Safer operations involve excising a length of Fallopian tube and ligating the ends, or cutting the tubes, ligating and then overlapping the stumps and ligating for a second time. These methods should be quick and bloodless. When the tube is sectioned the cut ends can be induced to undergo occluding fibrosis by burning with diathermy, crushing or injecting sclerosing solutions such as sodium morrhuate. In Irving's technique the middle third of the tube is ligated in two places with catgut and a length of tube excised. The proximal stump is then buried in a 1 cm incision in the uterine wall, just below the cornu, and the distal stump is buried between peritoneal layers of the broad ligament. Bleeding from the uterine incision can be difficult, especially if the operation is attempted at the time of a caesarean section. Cornual resection is another technique which involves cutting the uterus and in this the uterine end of the tube, together with part of the uterine wall, is removed, but it has a significant failure rate.

Bilateral salpingectomy is the most rational operation. It has the disadvantages of taking slightly longer, though not appreciably longer than Irving's procedure, and of involving the possibility of more bleeding, but it has the advantage of being very effective.

The ovarian and uterine arteries anastomose in the broad ligament and many small blood vessels pass to the Fallopian tubes in the mesosalpinx. Good haemostasis must be achieved whatever operation is undertaken.

It is possible to ligate the tubes through a vaginal approach and if a pelvic floor repair is being done it may be reasonable to combine this operation with a sterilization. However, the tubes are less accessible and it is more difficult to deal with emergencies such as unexpected bleeding. It is possible to mistake the round ligament for the tubes. Sterilizing operations can also be performed through a laparoscope.[7] A general anaesthetic is usually necessary but the operation requires little preparation, is brief and patients rarely require more than 60 hours in hospital and feel well on discharge. The innermost portion of the Fallopian tubes is coagulated using a diathermy and a limited follow-up of cases with a second laparoscopy shows complete cornual blockage and fibrosis for 2 cm. Adhesions and other complications have not been reported. The limitation of the method is that few surgeons are skilled in laparoscopy techniques. Transuterine electrocoagulation has also been attempted[8] but the failure rate is 1 in 10, or higher, and it cannot be recommended, although the technique might be open to improvement.

(c) OPERATIONS AT DELIVERY OR TERMINATION

Repeated caesarian sections are surgically difficult and present an increasing risk to the woman. Most surgeons offer sterilization at the third operation and it may be considered at the second in certain cases. It is also reasonable to consider sterilization when a caesarean section is performed for the first time in a woman who has had previous vaginal deliveries.

Sterilization after vaginal delivery is surgically straightforward. The uterus is large and the tubes readily accessible through a short abdominal incision made just inferior to the umbilicus. The operation can be performed within hours of delivery or two or three days later and, if the baby was delivered in hospital the operation does not require a separate admission. When doing a post partum sterilization in a woman with severe cardiac disease 10 to 14 days should elapse between delivery and the operation.

Abdominal hysterotomy can be combined with any suitable procedure for interrupting the Fallopian tubes. There is an increased failure rate if vaginal hysterotomy is combined with tubal ligation and Boyson and McRae[9] report five failures out of 26 with this method. It is probably better to choose an abdominal approach if it is known that sterilization is to be combined with termination.

(d) HYSTERECTOMY

It is not generally realized that hysterectomy can be an over-worked operation and it is sometimes performed for a series of confused and partially inadequate reasons, amongst which, if the case is reviewed honestly, excess fertility may be the most important. Reviewing 1,701 hysterectomy specimens received in a pathological department, Bieren and Hundley[10] found that 300 (18 per cent) were normal. There had been no gynaecological indication for the operation in 43 cases and only questionable indications in the remaining 197.

Confusion of thought is not uncommon in the realm of family planning and a woman may seek hysterectomy when she really needs to be sterilized and a surgeon may carry out the operation because he finds it easier to convince himself an organ is diseased and remove it, than to make a straightforward decision about tubal ligation. This is particularly likely with Roman Catholic doctors and patients and is a practice encouraged by the 1968 Papal Encyclical. As hysterectomy has a higher mortality than more conservative sterilizing procedures, and as the death rate exceeds that which would be justifiable on grounds of prophyllaxis against malignancy, the practice is to be condemned.

(e) RADIATION

Irradiation with radium or deep X-rays produces an artificial menopause and consequent sterility. The procedure is comparable to surgical castration, it carries the risk of inducing malignancy and has no place whatsoever in family planning.

SIDE EFFECTS

1 Biological

Tubal ligation is unassociated with any known change in female physiology. The ovarian cycle and menstruation continue unchanged. The unfertilized eggs are lost into the peritoneal cavity.

The woman who has been sterilized is still subject to the normal incidence of gynaecological disease and about 10 per cent of those who have had tubal ligation subsequently have a hysterectomy, pelvic floor repair or develop cancer. It has been argued that hysterectomy should replace tubal ligation but the higher mortality of the former procedure does not justify this claim.[11]

Following vasectomy sperm production and hormone output from the testicular interstitial cells continues normally. Macrophages (probably derived from the basal layer of the epithelium) accumulate in the epididymus and vas deferens and phagocytose the sperm that are produced. Nearly all the sperm are destroyed intraluminally but extravasation of sperm into the subepithelial tissues occurs on rare occasions.[12] Phagocytosis of sperm is a normal process in the male genital tract although, of course, the rate is greatly increased after vasectomy.

Antibodies to sperm can be demonstrated in a proportion of vasectomised men, but these appear to be of no significance and do not reduce the chance of restoring fertility if reanastomosis is attempted.[13] Roberts[14] has reported on six men who had a variety of unexplained disorders, usually involving hypoglycaemia, but it is difficult to evaluate these observations which were made in a practice where vasectomy is common and they require confirmation or refutation at a statistical level.

2   Surgical risks

(a) DEATH

A generation ago tubal ligation had a significant death rate rising to 1 per cent for post partum operations.[15] Today, many large series are without mortality or have a very low rate, such as one death in 1,055 post partum sterilizations.[4] A small minority of women are sterilized because of a medical condition, such as severe cardiac or renal disease, which makes pregnancy dangerous. It must be remembered that these cases also carry an increased risk of death at a sterilizing operation. Lull in 1940[16] recorded five deaths in 589 sterilizations and in all the fatal cases the women had a complicating illness.

The only deaths foreseeable after vasectomy appear to be complications of anaesthesia and infection.

(b) INFECTIONS AND OTHER COMPLICATIONS

About one woman in fifty is pyrexial after tubal ligation and one in thirty may have local wound infection. In the long term hydrosalpinges and adhesions may develop in one in twenty patients but these are usually asymptomatic.[4]

About one in fifty men develops a haematoma at the site of the vasectomy. A non-bacterial epididymitis sometimes occurs. Long-term surgical side effects, such as expulsion of non-absorbable ligatures, are rare and usually trivial but spermatic granuloma can form in the proximal stump, especially if the vas was tied but not cauterized.[17]

(b) PSYCHOLOGICAL

The incidence of dissatisfaction and regret after sterilizing operations is said to vary from 0 to 40 per cent among published follow-ups.

TABLE 12. *Sexual satisfaction after vasectomy* (73 cases)

	Much more	Little more	No change	Little less
(*a*) Husband				
Feeling of freedom and decreased inhibition	10	40	22	1
Satisfaction with coitus	6	49	15	3
(*b*) Husband's report on wife				
Feeling of freedom and decreased inhibition	13	14	15	1
Ability to reach climax	8	28	35	2

Clearly the nature of the sample, the cultural background, the length of time that has elapsed since the operation and the technique of evaluation all differ greatly.

Both sexes respond similarly to simple questions, such as 'Would you have the operation again?' 'Are you sorry you were sterilized?' and only 2 to 5 per cent report regret.[18, 19, 20] The great majority of men and women report unchanged or improved health after sterilizing operations and many have better marriages. In a follow-up of vasectomized men Ferber, Tietze and Lewit (table 12) found that 70 per cent claimed to be happier than before the operation and less than 2 per cent less happy. For many there is an improvement in their sexual life and, in the above study, mean coital frequency per month rose from 8·4 before the operation to 9·8 afterwards. Adams,[18] Lu and Chun[4] and Thomson and Baird,[21] in surveys of patient coming from very different cultural backgrounds, have reported similar findings in women after tubal ligation.

When careful psychiatric tests or semidirective interviews are used, up to 15 per cent of any sample followed up can be demonstrated to have some degree of dissatisfaction[22, 23] with the operation, but those who are most disturbed by sterilization are often men or women with a history of previous psychiatric instability.[24] There is no evidence that severe psychiatric disturbance after the operation is any higher than among the population as a whole, although dramatic cases, such as suicide shortly after sterilization, tend to make an undue impact on the medical as well as the lay mind. There is, however, a group of patients who, having obtained sterilization, will rapidly weave it into the fabric of their emotions. One such group of women has been described as having 'feelings of inferiority, weakness, emptiness, being torn up inside, and being a damaged changed person. They had convictions that many other structures, particularly sexual organs, had been involved and destroyed or injured in the operation. Many women reported a decrease in sexual desire and gratification, and associated this with being a "castrated woman". All subsequent misfortunes of life, accidents, obesity, frigidity, marriage failure, and new physical illness were blamed on the operation.'[22] Regret is less likely if the woman requested the operation than when the physician suggested it and less likely when it was done for reasons of family size than for organic disease or previous caesarean section.[21, 25] Sterilizing operations are more likely to have an unsatisfactory outcome if the couple were in disagreement about the need for operation: the two worst results in one follow-up occurred in the only four cases where the wife had disagreed with the husband's wish to be sterilized.[5] Sterilization is a powerful weapon which men and women can use to hurt others or themselves.

The details of adverse responses to sterilizing operations differ in the two sexes. In women there is sometimes an immediate reaction which may last several months. The woman may become overprotective towards her children, she may complain of 'dragging' pelvic pain or she may adopt illogical but revealing attitudes towards her marital life, such as limiting coitus to what was previously the fertile period. No doubt these changes in attitude also account for some of the menstrual disturbances and cases of secondary dysmenorrhea that are reported to follow tubal ligation.

Emotionally, it is very difficult for men to avoid equating vasectomy with castration, and using interviews and self-administered psychological tests Ziegler and his co-workers[26] in California have been able to demonstrate such an attitude among a number of vasectomized men, and the proportion rises among those who were psychologically unstable before the operation. It is revealing that only 50 per cent of men are willing for those around them to know they have been sterilized and less than one-third recommend the operation to other men.[5] It appears that vasectomy can stimulate fears of impotency and castration but all normal men adjust to these, although they may be left with a slight reluctance to impress their way of thinking on the outside world.

The fear that a sterilized couple may want more children because of family death or as a result of one partner remarrying is widespread, but in practice it is an unusual cause for regret. In over 800 tubal ligations only three women were dissatisfied with the operation because they wanted more children, and the likelihood of regret does not appear to be very strongly correlated with the parity or age of the patient.[22] Among 1,000 high parity women in Hongkong the problem arose once —and dissatisfaction with pregnancy following sterilizing failures was more common than a desire to have further children.[4]

Many side effects are culturally specific; for example, the Chinese believe sterilization makes the temper worse and affects the memory, and in the series quoted above between one-third and one-half of the women complained of these symptoms. Certain Roman Catholic patients may express guilt or bitterness after the operation, although it is interesting that in Switzerland the proportions of Catholic and Protestant women having tubal ligation corresponds exactly with those in the population at large[22] and subsequent regret at having been sterilized was in no way related to the woman's religion. There is no association between sterilization and marital infidelity: in 73 cases followed up by Ferber and others[5] only one man admitted increased extramarital intercourse after the operation and he had been having an affair before the vasectomy. The common response was that of a man who said, 'I think less about other women than I did, I guess it's because I'm more satisfied now.'

(d) FAILURES

Pregnancy has been recorded after subtotal hysterectomy and no sterilizing procedure is 100 per cent effective. Most epithelial tubes will recanalize after damage and the Fallopian tubes and vas deferens are no exception. In the case of female sterilization the skill and experience of the surgeon is almost as important as the technique adopted. In the case of vasectomy the physician's skill in handling the man and ensuring that he returns for follow-up examination is very significant and less surgical finesse is required.

The failure rate for tubal ligation is given in table 13: it is lowest with the more complex operations but for a given technique the junior staff have a higher failure rate than their seniors.[27] The failure rate also rises when tubal ligation is combined with some other operation (table 14). When pregnancy occurs after tubal ligation there is an increased risk of ectopic gestation involving the damaged area of Fallopian tube.

The failure rate after vasectomy is more difficult to evaluate because the patient may fail to take adequate contraceptive precautions during

TABLE 13. *Pregnancy after tubal ligation by method*

	Number in series	Pregnancies	%
Pomeroy	5,477	22	0·4
Madlener	7,829	113	1·4
Irving	1,056	0	0·0
Cornual resection	311	9	2·8

TABLE 14. *Pregnancy after tubal ligation by time and route*

	Number in series	Pregnancies	%
Abdominal tubal ligation	93	0	0·0
Hysterotomy and tubal ligation	77	1	1·3
Caesarian section and tubal ligation	418	14	3·3
Vaginal tubal ligation	38	2	5·2
Post partum (24 hours) tubal ligation	286	16	5·6

the post-operative interval of residual fertility. Thirty per cent of men still have viable sperm eight weeks after the operation. Schmidt[17] records five cases of genuine recanalization amongst 432 patients but claims that the number can be reduced by careful techniques.

REPAIR OF STERILIZING OPERATIONS

When deciding on a sterilizing operation the patient and doctor should regard it as irreversible, as only in this way can they make a valid decision. But if the situation subsequently arises in which a patient wishes to have his or her fertility restored the case should be looked at sympathetically and every effort made to meet the need.

Reversible operations, such as burying the Fallopian tube or ovary in the broad ligament have been tried in women but when there is a real possibility of reversing the operation there is a significant chance of failure, and if certainty as a sterilizing procedure is achieved then the likelihood of reversibility is remote.

Following vasectomy the cut ends of the vas become fibrosed for approximately 1 cm and on the proximal side of the ligature the patent lumen becomes dilated. The incidence of reversibility depends upon the experience of the surgeon, the technique used and, most important, the form of the original operation. Reanastomosis is only possible if the cut ends can be reapproximated. Some surgeons can achieve a high degree of success and the Phadkes,[28] operating in India, on a series of 76 men found sperm in the semen of 63 following reanastomosis and in 42 cases the wife became pregnant. A good surgical exposure is necessary, all fibrosed tissue must be excised and the patent ends joined with 6/0 arterial silk sutures on atraumatic needles. The two ends are splinted on a nylon thread which is left in place for eight days. Great care is needed, ophthalmic instruments are of use, the operation takes 2 to 3 hours and requires a general anaesthetic.

Reversible sterilization has been attempted by inserting silicone plugs in the vas but this technique is still in the experimental stage.

EVALUATION

Most sterilizations are performed on couples in their early thirties. The decision should be a joint one and the doctor should help the man and his wife decide which partner is to have the operation. It is regrettable that surgeons from two otherwise unrelated specialisms are involved in operations which have a common purpose. Vasectomy is simple, safe and effective but has the mild disadvantage of not being immediately effective. In contrast to tubal ligation it involves no measurable risk to life, it carries a reasonable chance of reversibility and it can be done as an outpatient procedure. When a normal, stable, happy couple requests sterilization vasectomy is preferable to tubal ligation. Tubal ligation involves opening the peritoneal cavity, it usually requires a general anaesthetic and the indications for performing the operation must be carefully considered.

Deaths and failures following female sterilization are of the same order of magnitude as those involved in the use of oral contraceptives. Most records of pregnancy following a sterilizing operation are made without reference to the interval since the operation so it is impossible to calculate failure per HWY. Sterilization is probably 5 to 20 times as effective as oral contraception, although this factor will be reduced for the sophisticated who use oral contraception well and increased for couples from the 'problem family' group. If a death rate of 1 in 5,000 is taken as representative of the mortality from female sterilization then the risks of this contraceptive technique approximate to 5 years use of oral contraceptives (using the higher mortality for oral contraceptives which is calculated on women over the age of 35).

The risks of the operation should be assessed slightly differently if the abdomen has been opened, although it must be remembered that sterilization adds slightly to the risk of caesarian section or termination and the operation is also marginally less effective at this time. Sterilization can be offered at caesarean section, or prolapse repair, and may be appropriate when a late abortion is done by hysterotomy (although there is never any justification in postponing abortion until such time as a hysterotomy may be indicated).

When sterilization is done at the time of delivery or termination the woman is often in hospital and usually highly motivated towards family planning. In many cases it is wise to combine tubal ligation and induced abortion. Some doctors however have the habit of presenting a package deal to the patient: 'I will terminate your pregnancy if you agree to be sterilized at the same time.' and *vindictiveness of this kind is a form of blackmail which should have no place in gynaecological practice.*[29]

The importance of sterilization, both for the individual and at a demographic level, is that it stops further pregnancies, but it is easy to overlook one of its main defects which is that for many people it comes too late in their reproductive life: in Barglow and Eisner's[22] analysis of tubal ligation in Switzerland 95 per cent of the women interviewed had not wanted the pregnancy preceding the operation; in Lu and Chun's[4] series in Hongkong the average parity was six, and in Thompson and Baird's series[21] more women regretted not being sterilized earlier than regretted having the operation. While the operation remains irreversible it is difficult to escape from this dilemma, but the pattern of reproduction in the Western world is now of a type where sterilization, if used intelligently, can be the contraceptive method of choice after two or three children and in relatively young couples.

If a couple considers their family complete then it is probably best to use oral contraceptives (or perhaps an IUD) for one or two years and then, if they remain of the same mind, sterilization is reasonable. The pattern of infant death is now such (figure 28) that after the first few months of life a child is a very secure member of the family, but as many infant deaths occur in the first 24 hours after delivery there are good reasons for delaying post partum sterilization for a couple of days.

Sterilization is the most negative and final form of contraception and in many ways it is remarkable that so many men and women express satisfaction with the operation on subsequent questioning. It is not illogical to believe that a contraceptive procedure has been the best choice without, at the same time, feeling enthusiastic about it. No procedure is perfect and family limitation, like respecting your neighbour's property or keeping certain hours of work, is an intrinsic and inescapable frustration of civilized living.

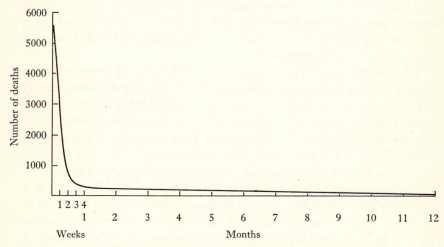

Fig. 28. The pattern of infant mortality, England and Wales 1966.

The doctor should avoid pressurizing a patient into having an operation and should be very cautious if he thinks husband and wife disagree on the subject. When one or both partners to a marriage are emotionally unstable then sterilization may prove a less satisfactory operation. Against this must be set the fact that a succession of unwanted pregnancies could have had an even more adverse effect on the couple and their existing children, especially as even a mild degree of psychological disturbance is often associated with poor use of patient-dependent methods of contraception.

Sterilization is becoming more acceptable but past attitudes linger on among both doctors and the general public: in Britain the operation is not offered as part of the National Health Service because it is considered difficult to justify as being in the direct medical interest of the patient rather than his family. In the United Kingdom and the United States social attitudes towards sterilization are more disparaging than towards, say, ovulation inhibition and the doctor's task is a dual one of helping his patients to see the operation rationally and of educating society as a whole.

13 ABORTION

The obstetric and legal definition of abortion is the termination of a pregnancy before the twenty-eighth week of gestation. In the eyes of the law a fetus is not viable before twenty-eight weeks of pregnancy, and it is only on rare occasions that fetuses delivered before the seventh month have been salvaged. Abortions may be either spontaneous or induced and induced abortions are subdivided into legal and illegal. The law relating to induced abortion is discussed in chapter 14.

Abortion is a subject of immense importance in the overall pattern of human fertility. In some modern urban communities induced abortions may account for one in two of all conceptions, and given an unfortunate combination of contraceptive ignorance and economic circumstances, they may outnumber live births. It is a neglected subject in medical education and practice.

INCIDENCE

1 Spontaneous

The incidence of spontaneous abortion is difficult to establish. There is a universal tendency to under-report abortions and a considerable pregnancy wastage takes place before a woman is aware conception has occurred. An unknown percentage of induced abortions may be passed off as spontaneous miscarriages.

One way of attempting to eliminate errors is to study women who have used contraceptive methods and then abandoned them to have a planned pregnancy. Tietze found that only 7 per cent in such a group had spontaneous abortions, but the survey may have missed some early abortions and have been biased towards women of a particular fertility and social class (figure 29). Most other surveys suggest that spontaneous abortion, taking place after pregnancy has been diagnosed, accounts for 10 to 20 per cent of pregnancies. In a prospective survey of Indian women 10·5 per cent of known conceptions ended in spontaneous abortions, and it was thought that some under-reporting was likely.[1] In most series of western women the spontaneous abortion rate has been put at about 15 per cent (figure 30). In a combined survey involving 6,844 women Shapiro, Jones and Densen[2] found an overall spontaneous fetal wastage of 14 per cent. The greatest loss was between two and four months of gestation. Women in the 20 to 24 age-group having their first pregnancy had fewest spontaneous abortions (8 per cent) and the maximum occurred in women over 35 having their fourth or subsequent pregnancy (20 per cent).

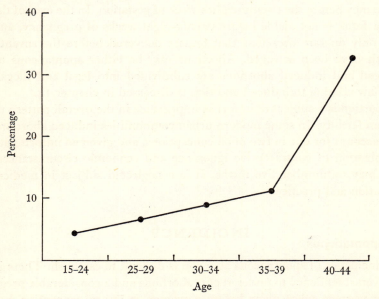

Fig. 29. Percentage of spontaneous abortions during 1,497 planned pregnancies

If spontaneous abortions occurring before the first missed period are included then the incidence is increased. Among the small series of human ova recovered during the early stages of human reproduction Hertig and Rock[3] estimate that 90 per cent remain viable at the late blastocyst stage, 58 per cent at implantation but only 42 per cent at the twelfth day after fertilization, and in a series of 28 embryos collected before the first missed period 12 were classified as abnormal and in 7 it was thought abortion would have taken place later. Among women carrying abnormal conceptuses previous spontaneous abortions are slightly more common (13 per cent) than in those with healthy ova (9 per cent).

There is evidence from the analysis of chromosome preparations that up to one-third of embryos aborted in the first trimester of pregnancy are abnormal. Autosomal trisomy, an easily recognized abnormality, is

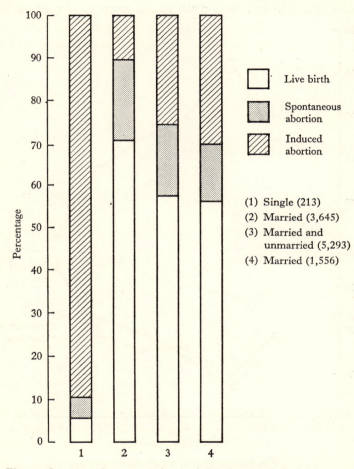

Fig. 30. Outcome of pregnancy in married and unmarried women.

found in 10 per cent of spontaneous abortions but in only 0·2 per cent of the general population.[4] It must be concluded that abnormalities of mammalian reproduction are common and that spontaneous abortion is an important regulatory mechanism which protects the species against an overwhelming number of congenitally abnormal offspring.

2   Induced Abortion

The incidence of induced abortion is even more difficult to determine than that of spontaneous abortion. Women do not readily confess to criminal abortions and these make up the majority of cases in Western

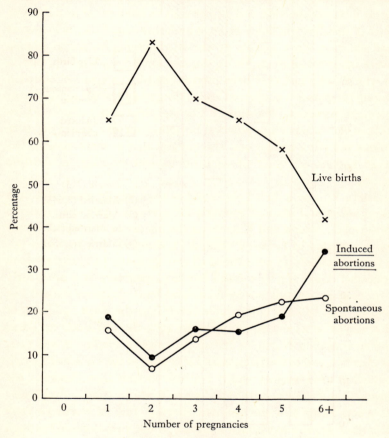

Fig. 31. Outcome of pregnancy by parity.

Europe and America. The situation is further complicated because the distribution of spontaneous and induced abortions is at many points parallel with respect to parity and age (figure 31). The frequency of induced abortions varies from community to community and nation to nation and it varies at different times within the same society. It is more common in urban than rural areas and the problem is aggravated in areas which are economically depressed either in relation to their previous condition, as in Western Europe in the late 1920s, or in relation to neighbouring countries, as in contemporary Eastern Europe today.

In a National Opinion Poll survey carried out in the United Kingdom in 1966, 4 per cent of women in a sample of over 2,000 admitted to having an induced abortion and 11 per cent to attempting to induce an abortion. This survey is likely to have underestimated the incidence of criminal abortion. In a sample of several thousand American women who were interviewed in depth by the late Dr Kinsey's group, one in five of women who had ever been married had had a criminal abortion and among pregnancies conceived and ending outside marriage nine out of ten ended in induced abortions.[5] The sample was not wholly representative of the American population but other surveys, based on more meticulous sampling techniques, also suggest that in many nations between 20 and 30 per cent of conceptions end in induced abortion (figure 30).

In Eastern Europe induced abortion has been legally obtainable on a variety of social and medical grounds for approximately ten years. In Czechoslovakia, Poland and Yugoslavia the incidence of hospital terminations has settled at between 30 and 35 abortions per hundred live births (approximately 25 per cent of all conceptions). In Hungary there is a universal desire for very small families, contraceptives are poorly used, ineffective methods predominate and legal abortions exceed live births (135 : 100).[6] Given comparable conditions this high incidence of abortion can arise in any community. In 1965 the birth rate in Turin and the surrounding Northern Italian province of Piedmont was 13·4, almost exactly equal to the Hungarian birth rate for the same year (13·1); contraceptives are even less readily available in Italy than Hungary, the marriage rate and age structure of the two societies are comparable, therefore it seems likely that the criminal abortion rate in Northern Italy parallels the legal rate in Hungary. Again, in one east London borough between 1924 and 1934 the birth rate fell from 18·2 to 13·2, while the number of hospital admissions for abortion doubled.[7]

CRIMINAL ABORTION

The techniques used for inducing criminal abortions vary. In the USA the private physician carries out over 80 per cent of abortions. In the United Kingdom self-induced abortions and lay operators play a larger role. Higginson's syringe with soap and water or Dettol has been and remains the most popular single method of producing a criminal abortion. Slippery elm, which swells when inserted in the cervix, the use of a catheter and knitting needles account for a smaller number of cases. Potassium permanganate crystals are sometimes placed in the vagina; they cause ulceration but usually leave the pregnancy intact. At least twice as many abortions are attempted as are carried through. A wide variety of 'female pills' is available and purchased as emmenogogues and abortifacients. They are sold by chemists, herbalists, and mail order firms and labelled as 'For irregularities, scanty and painful menstruation due to shock, colds, etc.' or as bringing 'swift and Blessed relief'. Cascara and iron salts are common constituents and their price is always grossly inflated. Most have no pharmacological basis for their alleged actions but contain ergot, quinine and certain antimitotic agents which, while uncertain as abortifacients, can poison or kill the pregnant woman or produce a grossly abnormal baby. Unfortunately, quinine is freely available without prescription and a considerable trade centres on its spurious claim to cure colds and cramps in old women and unwanted pregnancy in young. Toxic effects arise in doses in excess of about 4 g. There may be nausea, vomiting, abdominal pain, tinnitus, deafness, visual impairment, vertigo, hypotension, fever and convulsions and death. Blindness is due to a direct effect on the retina and to vasoconstriction and stellate ganglion block is a rational treatment.[8]

The dangers of criminal abortion are the immediate ones of haemorrhage, air or fluid embolism or intravascular haemolysis. Uterine perforation can occur. Sepsis is quite common and can be severe, especially if *Clostridium welchli* is present, and may lead to sterility or death. Before the introduction of antibiotics and blood transfusion between 1 and 2 per cent of the abortions admitted to hospital died. Today, deaths from abortion are much rarer. Deaths and complications are fewest when the criminal abortionist is medically qualified: only 2·8 per cent of Gebhard's series of American women having illegal abortions reported severe physical side effects.[5] Rhodes has estimated that the chances of dying from a criminal abortion are approximately twice those of dying from childbirth.[9] In England and Wales (1963) 239 women died from delivery and the complications of childbirth, that is 2·6 per cent of all the deaths among women in the 15 to 44 age-group and 49 died from abortion (spontaneous and criminal), that is 0·5 per cent of all deaths.

Roman Catholics and those associated with the medical profession have a higher than average incidence of abortion and negroes and some lower socio-economic groups a below average frequency.

ABORTION AND FAMILY PLANNING

Most legal and criminal abortions are performed for social reasons. When the social or economic pressures for small families are strong, couples will resort to whatever methods of family limitation are available. During the evolution of birth control practices in urban societies there appears to be a phase when the incidence of both contraception and abortion rises. This is probably the pattern in much of Latin America today. Ineffective and inappropriate methods of contraception and induced abortion may be found side by side. However, improvements in contraception still take place in a community where abortion is freely available; for example, in Hungary there has been a rise in the use of the condom (17 to 25 per cent) and diaphragm (4 to 12 per cent) at a time when there has been no restriction on legal abortion.[6]

In Britain and the United States there is a widespread resort to contraception and the induced abortion rate is lower than in most countries. However, the situation is still open to improvement and recent falls in the birth rate may have been associated with a jump in the abortion rate.

INDICATIONS

1 Social

Social and medical factors are closely interwoven in the field of abortion. In England the law relating to abortion was changed in 1967 and allows the woman's 'total environment' to be taken into account. While not permitting termination on purely social grounds it allows a decision for mixed medico-social reasons. An attempt is being made to allow a humane consideration of social factors in the redrafting of some American state laws.

When a country passes a liberalizing law on abortion the pressure of social indications soon manifests itself. The Swedish law on abortion was changed in 1938 and at that time there were less than 500 legal terminations a year, over three-quarters of which were for medical reasons. By 1953 there were 4,915 abortions, of which only 35 per cent were for strictly medical indications. The nations of Eastern Europe have gone furthest in legalizing abortion for social reasons. Their experience is probably representative of any urban, industrialized society. Social indications account for at least 90 per cent of legal abortions in Czechoslovakia, 94 per cent in Slovenia, 96 per cent in Hungary and 99 per cent of cases in Rumania.[6]

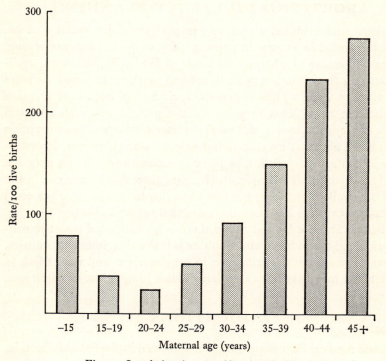

Fig. 32. Legal abortion rate (Czechoslovakia, 1961).

(a) THE MOTHER

About half the women having induced abortions, if questioned concerning their reasons, say they already have as many or more children than they feel able to cope with, between 10 and 20 per cent mention limitations imposed by finanial reasons; about 15 per cent report they are unmarried and amongst the remainder a wide variety of reasons such as the death or invalidism of the husband, rape, carnal knowledge, alcoholism, etc. is offered. The incidence of induced abortion rises with age and parity. When the induced abortion rate is considered for different age-groups (figure 32) it is those at the extremes of reproductive life who have the most terminations: the very young who are mostly nulli-

parous and unmarried and the older women with several children. However, those with the highest abortion rates only make up a minority of
the total number having terminations.

Women refused a legal abortion commonly seek to terminate their
pregnancies elsewhere. For example, in one study in Sweden 68 out of
194 women refused a legal abortion failed to deliver at term,[10] and in
Prague 254 out of 555 women had criminal or spontaneous abortions.
When a woman is driven to seek an abortion by pressure of social
circumstances she deserves objective and sympathetic advice. It is of the
utmost importance that a women with an unwanted pregnancy should
turn for medical help as early as possible in pregnancy. The doctor who
gives intolerant or unrealistic advice may soon cease to be troubled by
requests for termination but he will have done so by sidestepping a great
mass of human misery and potential ill health. The issue must be faced
squarely and every possibility, from abortion through to adoption or
bringing in social services, considered. Under these circumstances some
pregnancies which might have ended in back-street abortions will be
carried to term. Whatever the outcome of the pregnancy it is imperative
to offer adequate contraceptive advice.

(b) THE CHILD

Children born to women refused abortions are at a disadvantage when
compared with children born to mothers who never sought a termination during pregnancy. In Sweden, Forssman and Thume[10] followed up
all those women in the city of Gottenborg whose application for a legal
termination was rejected between 1939 and 1941. The pregnancies that
went to term were paired with the next child of the same sex born in
the same hospital or township. The social and economic parameters of
the two groups of children matched well. Events which were open to
some degree of objective measurement were followed up (table 15) and
the authors conclude: 'the unwanted children were worse off in every
respect...the differences were often statistically significant, and when
they were not, they pointed in the same direction—to a worse lot for
the unwanted children. One may assume that the children who were not
born because their mothers got authorization for abortion would have
had to face still greater disadvantages socially and medically.' Perhaps
the saddest thing to note is the way in which the child of an unwanted
pregnancy tends to grow up into a boy or girl who marries early and has
more than an average number of children: undoubtedly many of these,

TABLE 15. *Follow-up of children born to women refused legal termination of pregnancy*

	Children born to women refused legal abortions (120)	Control group (120)	Statistical probability
Attended psychiatric clinic	34	18	0·01
Delinquency	22	10	0·05
Drunken misconduct	19	13	0·5
Public assistance	17	3	0·001
Educationally subnormal, attended special schools, etc.	13	6	0·1
Proceeded to higher education	17	40	0·001
University	5	11	(not sig.)
Unfit for military service	60	4	0·1
Married before 21	20	14	(not sig.)
Divorced	2	0	
Girls having children before age 21	14	7	

in their turn, are unwanted. In some ways it is remarkable that differences between the two groups should have become apparent at all, as the women in question had, in the opinion of their original assessors, insufficient grounds for termination. Many of the pregnancies must have been subject to the normal evolution of emotions in a pregnant woman and have been regarded as wanted babies at the time of birth. Conversely, the control group must have included a proportion of 'unwanted' conceptions even if their mothers never felt desperate enough to seek a legal abortion.

(c) THE UNMARRIED

One of the distinguishing features of the Gottenborg series was the raised incidence of illegitimacy, parental separation, adoption and fostering among children born to women refused abortions (table 16). When assessing the social indications for abortion among the unmarried, and especially among the teenage unmarried, it is important to remember that the choice is often between abortion, forced marriage or adoption and the opportunity for the adolescent single girl to keep and rear her child rarely arises. Immediate problems of pregnancy, labour and the puerperium may not present as many emotional problems as might be

TABLE 16. *Background of children born to women refused legal termination of pregnancy*

	Children born to women refused legal abortions	Control
Born out of wedlock	32	9
Never legitimized	27	4
Adopted	8	0
Reported for unsatisfactory home conditions	17	6
Child removed from home by local authorities	2	0
Foster home	19	4
Children's home	30	10
Parents divorced before child age 15	23	13

imagined, but the long-term consequences for the child, if born, and for the mother must not be overlooked. Marriage following unwanted teen-age pregnancy has a poor outlook: further education is usually curtailed for the mother and often for the father as well and divorce is three to four times as common as among couples who marry and conceive under twenty.

2 Psychiatric

Admissions to psychiatric hospitals are significantly in excess of the expected number during the months following delivery although there is a reduction during pregnancy itself.[11] The young, and women approaching the end of their reproductive lives, are most at risk and depression and mania are the commonest diagnoses.

More controversy centres around the psychiatric indications for abortion than practically any other topic in medicine. In many countries, and until 1968 in British practice, the picture has been complicated and distorted by laws linking termination to situations constituting a mental or physical threat to a woman's life. It is true that there can never be a complete divorce of psychiatric and social factors but equally obvious that psychiatrists have been called upon to give opinions in cases where termination was being performed on primarily social or humanitarian grounds. The debate now polarizes around two points well summarized by Donnelly (1958): 'As medical men I believe we should definitely confine our indications for therapeutic abortion to strictly medical reasons. We should be doctors of medicine, not socio-economic prophets' and Lidz (1958): 'let us be frank about this. When the psychiatrist says that there is a suicidal risk, in many instances he does not mean that at all, but feels that there are strong socio-economic grounds for a therapeutic abortion. Since the only grounds for abortion in many states is if it is felt that there is a threat of death, suicidal risk is thus established as the only legal way out of the situation.' There are those who would restrict termination to psychiatric conditions which have been precipitated or aggravated by the pregnancy and which can be relieved only by abortion, but few conditions fulfil these criteria and some would maintain that there are none. Others will base their decisions on broader grounds, considering the mother as the most indispensable member of the family group, and attempting to assess the effects of the pregnancy on existing children and the consequences of the mother's illness on the potential child. Yet others will consider the immediate health of the mother as of paramount importance and place less emphasis on the long-term course of the woman's condition. Whatever criteria are accepted, it must be remembered that psychiatry is an inexact branch of medicine and therapy, including termination, may be disappointing in its results. When advising a woman with any psychiatric condition on termination it should be remembered that the early weeks of pregnancy are a brief episode in the whole cycle of human reproduction, which may be said to begin when the germ cells are set aside during intrauterine life and to be still unended when the elderly are baby-sitting for their grandchildren. The responsibility of forcing a pregnancy to continue in a woman who, for example, is a psychopath or a schizophrenic (perhaps of such severity as to have necessitated a leucotomy) may be as great or greater than that of terminating the pregnancy.

(a) REACTIVE DEPRESSION (AFFECTIVE PSYCHOSIS)

This is the commonest condition to present for consideration regarding termination. There is an exaggerated emotional response to the pregnancy: crying, threats of suicide, sleeplessness, self guilt and self deprecation and occasionally delusions may be present. There may be a history of instability in childhood, of previous mental breakdown, of previous puerperal psychosis and a family history of mental disease.

Some reactive depressions improve during the latter part of pregnancy and most lift after delivery. The possibility of long-term illness is not high and during pregnancy it is difficult to predict the likelihood of puerperal psychosis after delivery.[12] It is possible to carry a woman with reactive depression to term given sufficiently intense support and the possibility of continuous hospital care. Some physicians have even resorted to electroconvulsive therapy, but the immediate anguish of the mother usually justifies termination. Although no specific follow-up has been conducted on the children born to mothers who have been carried through a reactive depression in pregnancy, the long-term effects are likely to be as bad or worse than those of other unwanted children.

(b) ENDOGENOUS DEPRESSION

Pregnancy may occur in the course of an endogenous depression or the depression may supervene or be precipitated by the pregnancy, but the progress of the disease is not likely to be greatly altered by termination. Whatever the outcome of the pregnancy the woman may need intensive care.

(c) SUICIDE AND THREATS OF SUICIDE

Suicide among pregnant women has been a card in the hand of both the proponents and opposers of abortion law reform, often ceasing to be the subject of rational argument. Some doctors maintained that practically every women with an unwanted pregnancy was a suicide risk, but now they have been overtrumped by the demonstration that suicide is less common in pregnant women than in the population as a whole. In 1953 the suicide rate among women aged 14 to 50 in New York was 5·5/100,000. The incidence of suicide among pregnant women was 0·55/100,000.[13] Unfortunately, these facts have sometimes been presented the other way round, namely that a pregnant woman never commits suicide as a result of the stress of an unwanted pregnancy. This is false (and has been the cause of at least one preventable death[14]) and between 3 and 5 per cent of women who commit suicide are pregnant.[15]

(d) PREVIOUS HISTORY OF PUERPERAL PSYCHOSIS

It is common for puerperal psychosis to recur. Martin,[16] working in St Patrick's Hospital, Dublin, followed up 75 women who had had puerperal psychosis and found one in five relapsed in the first subsequent pregnancy, and 13 per cent in the second. The overall recurrence rate for all subsequent pregnancies was nearly 19 per cent.

(e) SCHIZOPHRENIA

Women with established schizophrenia have a slightly below average birthrate, probably because they tend to spend part of their lives in institutional care. There is a lack of reliable information on the effect of pregnancy on the natural course of schizophrenia. It is not unreasonable to suggest that contrary decisions may be appropriate in different individual cases: pregnancy may lead to a remission and so may therapeutic termination. Probably the majority of cases are not grossly affected by the pregnancy, but a history of deterioration in previous pregnancies suggests a serious prognosis.

If a schizophrenic woman seeks an abortion her case must be looked at individually, wisely, humanely and on its merits. Often the decision to terminate will depend as much upon the doctor's assessment of the woman's capacity as a mother, or the possible consequences of another pregnancy on the established family, as on the effect of the pregnancy on the woman's psychiatric conditions.

(f) ANXIETY STATE AND HYSTERIA

These conditions seldom present indications for termination unless they are accompanied by depression.

(g) MANIC DEPRESSION, PSYCHOPATHIC PERSONALITY AND MENTAL DEFECT

As in schizophrenia, pregnancy may have little effect on the course of the disease, but the mother's capacity to be an adequate mother may be in question or a child, or additional child, may cause the breakdown of the family unit. The strain of a pregnancy, or additional pregnancy, may cut the uncertain ground from under a woman of subnormal intelligence who has previously fulfilled her role in society.

(h) GIRLS UNDER 16

Most societies recognize that girls under 16 years of age are immature and make sexual intercourse with someone of this age illegal. To carry a pregnancy to completion in the very young may well interrupt the whole long-term emotional development of the girl.

3 Eugenic

As the health of the community improves, congenital malformations become a relatively more important cause of illness. In the 1958 Perinatal Mortality Survey in Britain congenital diseases accounted for 17 per cent of stillbirths and 22 per cent of deaths in the first week of life.[17] The overall incidence of recognizable abnormalities at birth is 1·8 per

100 total births and the number rises if abnormalities which become apparent later in infancy are added (2·3 per cent).[18]

Many abnormalities are minor and do not impair the quality of human life. Some can be helped by palliative treatment but the severely handicapped child has little chance of fulfilment in life. When a congenital defect can be predicted then contraception and, where necessary, abortion must be considered.

A defective child may absorb all a woman's powers of motherhood and be a barrier to further pregnancies: abortion and a fresh start can secure more than one healthy child in the future. In a group of 120 children with neurological defects one-third of the mothers said they did not want any more children and a further fifth were cautious about future pregnancies.[19] Usually the birth of the child brought the parents together but some children went unaccepted or caused parental quarrels and a small number of cases led to the breakdown of marriage.

The fear of producing a defective child is one that faces every pregnant woman. If her fears have a basis in reality then they may become an overwhelming terror and abortion for the sake of the mother may also become necessary.

(a) GENETIC

If there is a family history of genetic abnormality or if an abnormal child has been born the parents will require skilled advice. Many diseases have a complex pattern of inheritance involving specialist knowledge and nearly all cases require reference to a clinic for genetic counselling.[20]

When an individual carrying an autosomal dominant marries a normal person, on average, half the children of the marriage will carry the disease. Those who do not have the disease will, when they in turn marry, have normal children. Some dominant conditions, for example achondroplasia, often appear as the result of a new mutation and when this occurs the remaining children of the family will not be at any added risk. Recessive conditions only become apparent when both parents carry the recessive gene. If one affected child has been born there is a one in four chance that the next child will be affected as well. Deleterious recessive genes are relatively common, and of course the normal siblings of an affected child will be heterozygous for the condition but the chances of marrying another person with the same recessive trait are very remote. Nearly all sex-linked genes are carried on the X chromosome. When a mother carries an X-linked disease, on average, one in two of her sons

TABLE 17. *Some examples of inherited disease*

Dominant conditions	Recessive conditions
achondroplasia	amaurotic family idiocy
acute intermittent porphyria	congenital adrenal hyperplasia
dystrophia myotonia	cystic fibrosis of the pancreas
Ehlers-Danlos syndrome	epidermolysis bullosa dystrophia
Huntington's chorea	galactosaemia
Marfan's syndrome (arachnodactyly)	glycogen storage disease
multiple exostoses	infantile progressive muscular
multiple polyposis of colon	atrophy (Werdnig-Hoffmann)
multiple telangiectasia	juvenile progressive muscular atrophy
myotonia congenita	metachromatic leucodystrophy
osteogenesis imperfecta	phenylketonuria
tuberose sclerosis	sickle cell anaemia
von Recklinghausen's disease	thalassaemia major (congenital
(multiple neurofibromatosis)	microcytosis)

X-linked conditions	Conditions with more than one type of inheritance
Christmas disease	gargoylism
haemophilia	muscular dystrophy
nephrogenic diabetes insipidus	retinitis pigmentosa

TABLE 18. *Approximate risk for subsequent children if one child is affected*

anencephaly	1 in 20
congenital malformations of heart	1 in 50
diabetes (onset under 30 years)	1 in 20
harelip and cleft palate	1 in 30
Hirchsprung's disease	1 in 20 (♂), 1 in 100 (♀)
mongolism	1 in 70
spina bifida cystica	1 in 20

will have the disease and one in two of her daughters will be carriers. Table 17 lists some inherited diseases which might require consideration for termination of pregnancy, if the mother wishes it.

The inheritance of some congenital diseases is very complex but the approximate empirical risk of recurrence can be given (table 18).

Incest presents a particular genetic problem, the offspring of father–daughter, son–mother, and brother–sister unions have 25 per cent of their autosomal genes in common. More than half such children may be mentally or physically handicapped.[21] The children of other, more remote, consanguineous relationships also appear to be at a disadvantage.

Intelligence is lower, although the interpretation of the correlations is complicated by the fact that people of low intelligence enter into inbred unions more commonly than others.[22] In cousin marriages the risk of congenital disease is twice that of unrelated spouses.

(b) TERATOGENICAL AGENTS

The risk of damage due to teratogenic agents can, by its very nature, only be predicted after pregnancy has commenced. It is the one situation in which adequate contraception will never eliminate the need for induced abortion. Unhappily, the chances of teratogenic damage may increase as the human environment becomes more complex and artificial.

(i) *Viral agents*

Rubella. An association between congenital malformations and German measles in the first trimester of pregnancy was noted by Gregg in 1941. The relationship has now been analysed and reviewed many times and, although there is some variation in the incidence of defect in different series, the overall picture is well established (figure 33).[23] In women contracting rubella before the twelfth week the commonest defects are heart disease (7 per cent), cataract (5·5 per cent) and deafness (2·5 per cent) but mental defect and pyloric stenosis are also slightly more common than in controls.[42]

The most dangerous time to have the disease is between the fifth and eighth week of pregnancy (figure 34). The embryo is unable to respond with a normal inflammatory reaction, cellular damage can be detected in many abortion specimens and the virus can persist for a long time and possibly beyond delivery. (New born babies with rubella embryopathies may infect those who look after them.) Live born infants have a lower birth weight and an infant mortality rate which is three times as high as that of children born to normal mothers. Many children exposed to rubella in the first trimester of pregnancy die before the age of two. When followed up over eight years or more the children who survive make a reasonable social adjustment and 92 per cent attend normal schools.[24]

German measles sometimes presents difficulties of diagnosis in adults but serological methods of confirming recent infection are available. Gamma-globulin prepared from rubella convalescents (obtainable from Blood Transfusion Centres) may be given to non-immune pregnant women if exposed to infection. Ordinary γ-globulin can be used instead

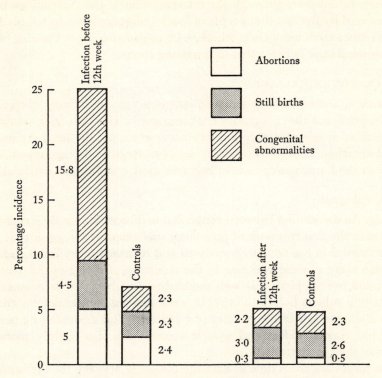

Fig. 33. Outcome of pregnancies complicated by rubella (578 cases).

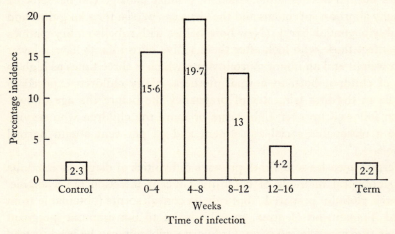

Fig. 34. Incidence of major malformations in pregnancies complicated by rubella.

but must be given in high doses (1,500 mg) as not all adults carry measles antibodies. The best prophyllaxis is exposure to the disease before puberty and avoidance of contacts during pregnancy.

Other viral diseases. An increasing number of viral diseases are being suspected of producing congenital defects but the risks are small and do not justify termination. Influenza in the first trimester of pregnancy may be associated with an increase of the fetal abnormality rate[25] but further work on this subject is necessary. Chickenpox (varicella) may cause chromosome abnormalities but no significant rise in the incidence of congenital defect, abortion or stillbirth was detected in a prospective study of nearly 300 pregnancies.[23] Endocardial fibroelastosis, presenting in infancy as cardiomegaly with heart failure, has been associated with mumps infection in the first trimester of pregnancy.[26] The evidence rests on a cutaneous sensitivity reaction and the risk is probably slight as, again, prospective studies have shown no easily measurable rise in congenital malformations.[27] Measles (morbilli), coxsackie infections, yellow fever, Bornholm disease and toxoplasmosis are also suspected of being teratogenic, but the evidence comes mainly from the study of individual cases and prospective studies have either not been attempted or have proved negative.

Variola can give rise to intrauterine infection leading to abortion, congenital defect or neonatal death and, if at all possible, vaccination and re-vaccination should be avoided during pregnancy.

(ii) *Drugs*

Thalidomide is the best known teratogenic drug and although it has been withdrawn from pharmacological use, its history and the pathogenesis of its effects are important. Some teratological agents vary in their actions on different species and despite the more rigorous testing of drugs which has evolved in recent years, fresh disasters of the thalidomide type are possible. In addition, there is an increasingly widespread use of new chemicals in industry and domestic life.

Thalidomide (α-phthalimidoglutarimide) was synthesized in 1956 and widely used as a hypnotic until November 1961 when evidence of its association with limb deformities became clearly apparent. Over 300 affected children were born in England and probably 3,000 in Germany. Its sale was never permitted in the United States.

Thalidomide proved most dangerous when taken between four and eight weeks of pregnancy and affected up to 20 per cent of babies at risk.

In addition to limb abnormalities, ear, eye, kidney and alimentary deformities were reported. It may even have acted before pregnancy in certain cases and indeed in animals it has been shown to produce damage to the blastocyst when given to the male before mating.

LSD. Drugs that are not available therapeutically, but are taken illicitly, present a risk which is virtually impossible to control at its source. LSD (lysergic-acid diethylamide) is known to cause chromosomal damage and cases of congenital malformation have been reported in women exposed to the drug.

Aminopterin (4-aminopteroylglutamic acid) is chemically related to thalidomide and was known to be teratogenic before the latter was marketed. It has a justified reputation as an abortifacient and is sometimes used by women attempting illegal abortions. If abortion fails there is a risk of inducing a bizarre syndrome of mental defect, poorly formed skull and lower jaw, low-set ears and limb abnormalities[28] and surgical termination is indicated (see also p. 200).

Miscellaneous. Carbon monoxide poisoning, due to attempted suicide early in pregnancy, is known to cause cerebral defect.[29]

A variety of drugs and chemicals produce fetal damage in experimental rats, for example meprobromate impairs the intelligence of the offspring of a treated mother, but on the whole the evidence demonstrates the need for cautious prescribing to pregnant women rather than abortion. Tetracyclines cross the placenta and are concentrated in the fetal skeleton and abnormalities have been recorded following very high doses, but the risks are small and should be non-existent when the drug is used properly. Sulphonamides and salicylates can be teratological in some species but appear harmless in man.

Most antimitotic drugs can kill or deform the embryo, but fortunately they are not likely to be given to pregnant women unwittingly, although termination should be considered if the father was taking a drug in this class before or at the time of fertilization.

(iii) *Radiation*

Both the maturing germ cells and the developing embryo are vulnerable to radiation damage. X-rays may be used diagnostically or therapeutically, α-, β-, and γ-rays may come from the local treatment of pelvic malignancy or the use of intravenous isotopes.

The fetus is probably about five times as sensitive to radiation as the adult. There is no evidence that there is any 'threshold' dose in the case of teratological damage and all sources of radiation, at least to the pelvis, must be avoided in pregnancy. The most radio-sensitive phase is the first 40 days of gestation and at this time neurological damage may follow routine pelvic X-ray and doses of 40 rad can produce serious defects. Radiation in excess of 200 rad 'will almost certainly result in fetal abnormality'.[30]

Minimal doses of X-rays may have other than teratological effects. Mahon[31] showed on a study of nearly three-quarters of a million children that the cancer mortality rate in children X-rayed in utero is 40 per cent greater than in the rest of the population. Mutations may be induced in the germ cells of the embryo which may not be apparent until the next generation or, if recessive, may not appear for several generations.

(iv) *Rhesus incompatibility*

If the husband is homozygous rhesus positive and previous babies have been severely affected, and the mother does not wish to risk a further pregnancy, then abortion is indicated. In cases of hydrops fetalis there is an increased risk of pre-eclamptic toxaemia, abruptio placentae and hypofibrinoginaemia at delivery which may add to the reasons for considering termination.

The incidence of rhesus incompatibility may be expected to decline now that sera are available to remove fetal red cells at delivery and, in addition, some affected babies can be saved by intrauterine transfusion.

(*c*) DIAGNOSIS

Cells can be cultured from the extra embryonic membranes for the analysis of chromosomes. When these techniques are perfected and readily available they will be applied in cases where a risk of abnormality exists and allow the diagnosis of certain types of deformity at a sufficiently early stage for therapeutic abortion to be performed.

In the longer term it may become practical to control fertilization in vitro and to select healthy eggs at the pre-implantation stages of development.

4 Medical

Fortunately the number of medical reasons for terminating a pregnancy decreases yearly. Jeffcoate[32] found that fewer than two pregnancies in 1,000 required termination on strictly medical grounds.

The recommendations of the Joint Paediatric and Obstetric Committee of the Tuberculosis Council are an appropriate foundation for considering all medical indications for abortion. They suggested the possibility of termination when the woman's health was seriously impaired by the disease, when she was psychologically disturbed at the prospect of pregnancy in association with her medical condition or when her condition was likely to be aggravated by the care of another child.

A woman whose health may be endangered by pregnancy deserves specialist care and advice concerning the actual risks. It is imperative that effective and appropriate contraceptive advice is offered (sterilization may be required) and if an unplanned pregnancy occurs, abortion must be seriously considered. Induced abortion must always be performed as early as possible in pregnancy.

(a) HEART DISEASE

Between 2 and 3 per cent of pregnant women have heart disease (defined as a diastolic murmur, cardiac enlargement or arrhythmia). Between 5 and 10 per cent of these cases come to termination.[33] Abortion is nearly always indicated if there has been an episode of heart failure in a preceding pregnancy.

(i) *Rheumatic*

Valvular disease, consequent on rheumatic fever, constitutes over 90 per cent of cardiological problems complicating pregnancy and accounts for about one-third of terminations taking place for medical reasons. Over the past thirty years the maternal mortality from this cause has fallen from 1 in 20 to 1 in 200. Nevertheless the decline has not been as marked as in other branches of obstetrics and the current death rate cannot be regarded as insignificant. Of the 1,410 maternal deaths in 1952–4 in the United Kingdom, 121 were due to cardiac lesions. Deaths occur at or after delivery and are mostly associated with pulmonary oedema.

Mitral stenosis is the predominant lesion in two-thirds of cases. Valvotomy can be performed in pregnancy but carries a mortality (over 5 per cent) which is greater than that of conservative obstetric care. Pregnancies occurring in patients who have had successful valvotomies present little risk. When a wanted pregnancy occurs in a woman whose rheumatic heart disease is associated with considerable disability (grade 3—moderate exertional intolerance, and grade 4—symptoms persisting at rest in bed) the possibility of termination followed by valvotomy may require review.

(ii) *Congenital*

More and more women with congenital heart disease are surviving to the reproductive years. The risks of pregnancy vary considerably (see table 19). Women with surgically repaired congenital heart lesions should be advised carefully and referred for specialist advice concerning the risks of pregnancy. Some repairs, for example resection of coarctation, are not without danger.

TABLE 19. *Maternal mortality in cases of congenital heart disease*

	No cases	Deaths (%)
Eisenmenger syndrome	37	27
Coarctation of aorta	232	4
Fallot's tetralogy	71	4
Ventricular septal defect	187	3
Atrial septal defect	261	2
Patent ductus arteriosus	318	0·5
Pulmonary stenosis	122	0

(iii) *Other heart diseases*

Chronic hypertension, if associated with renal or myocardial damage, may justify abortion. Malignant hypertension rarely afflicts women under 40. Pregnancy hastens the progress of the disease for the mother, the fetus has little chance of survival and termination is indicated. Coronary heart disease is virtually unknown in the child-bearing years.

(b) LUNG DISEASES

(i) *Pulmonary hypertension*

This may follow mitral stenosis, congenital heart disease, emphysema or arise without obvious cause. It is a rare but dangerous condition and between a third and a half of pregnant women with the condition die.[34]

(ii) *Pulmonary tuberculosis*

Abortion is rarely necessary, the problem only arising if there is gross impairment of lung function or some other criterion of the Tuberculosis Council is fulfilled. If pneumonectomy has been carried out and the patient has returned to leading a tolerably normal life pregnancy should not present an undue hazard.[35] If the disease has only recently become quiescent, PAS and isoniazid may be given during the last trimester of pregnancy and for some while after delivery. There is no evidence of any antituberculosis drug causing fetal damage.

(iii) *Other lung diseases*

Bronchiectasis, kyphoscoliosis and radical lung surgery, if they grossly impair the vital capacity, may be reasons for abortion, although women whose ventilating capacity has been halved can be brought safely to term.[36]

(c) OTHER DISEASES AFFECTED BY PREGNANCY

(i) *Kidney disease*

Bilateral hydronephrosis and bilateral pyelonephritis, if unassociated with hypertension, are compatible with carrying a wanted pregnancy to term. Pregnancy, by interfering with ureteric drainage, may make kidney infections more difficult and resistant to treatment by antibiotics. Termination is indicated in acute renal tuberculosis in order to prevent the disease spreading to the other kidney. The diseased kidney can be removed later.

Chronic nephritis complicates approximately one in 2,000 pregnancies. The mother can be carried to term but there is an appreciable fetal loss. Abortion is usually indicated if the glomerula filtration rate is reduced by 30 per cent or more and the blood pressure is raised. The woman should also be sterilized.

(ii) *Diabetes mellitus*

Pregnancy is thought to have an adverse effect on the long-term course of diabetes and is unwise in a woman who has a moderate to severe diabetic nephropathy or retinopathy. Abortion is also indicated if there has been repeated fetal loss or toxaemia in previous pregnancies. The availability of medical care and the parity of the woman should also be taken into account.[37]

Well treated with diligent antenatal care and hospital delivery the maternal mortality for diabetics is between 1 and 3 per cent. About one-third (range 10 to 40 per cent) of the babies of diabetic mothers die in utero or shortly after delivery. While a wanted pregnancy in a diabetic woman is a reasonable proposition it is neither humane nor safe to force a diabetic woman to continue an unwanted pregnancy. Sterilization should be considered if termination is performed.

There are also eugenic indications for abortion if there is a family history of the disease.

(iii) *Malignant conditions*

Cancer of the breast is exacerbated by pregnancy and termination is virtually imperative. Carcinoma of the cervix complicates approximately 1 in 2,000 pregnancies, its progress is worsened by pregnancy and a Wertheim hysterectomy should be performed. If the uterus is too large to permit a Wertheim hysterectomy the alternative is to do a hysterotomy followed by hysterectomy some days later. If the diagnosis is made late in pregnancy it may be possible to postpone the operation until the child is viable, but the risks are great.

Pregnancy is rarely complicated by other malignant diseases. Leukaemia and Hodgkin's disease are sometimes found but there is no firm evidence that pregnancy alters the prognosis of either. Abortion may be indicated on social or humanitarian grounds and in the case of Hodgkin's disease one in ten babies will be affected by the condition.

(iv) *Phaeochromocytoma*

When this complicates pregnancy it carries a mortality of over 50 per cent and abortion should be carried out.

(v) *Otosclerosis*

This is worsened by pregnancy in the majority of cases. Usually, although not in all women, the deafness reverts to the pre-pregnant state after delivery. Abortion is often recommended except for mild cases.

(vi) *Obstetric and gynaecological conditions*

In a developed country there are very few obstetric or gynaecological indications for therapeutic abortion, although some surgeons prefer to inflate trivial reasons rather than face the problem of social and medico-social indications squarely.[30] A history of difficult labours, or of a previous pelvic floor repair or of a vaginal fistula are all indications for caesarean section rather than termination of pregnancy.

Sometimes a history of severe pre-eclampsia, especially if it develops before 32 weeks of pregnancy, or of eclampsia may be an indication for abortion. *Chorea gravidarium* usually manifests itself in the first trimester of pregnancy and often the woman has a history of chorea or rheumatic fever (in many cases with valvular lesions). If the condition is progressive, or if the movements become violent, continuous, cause loss of sleep or are uncontrolled by sedatives then abortion is indicated. The disease can be fatal and termination must be performed before coma or delirium occur.

(d) INCAPACITATING DISEASES

Disseminated sclerosis, epilepsy, myasthenia gravis, ulcerative colitis and other physically incapacitating diseases are not, as far as is known, altered by pregnancy. But the care of a child or of another child may overstrain the mother and, while every medical and social support must be given to the woman with a wanted pregnancy, a woman with an unwanted pregnancy should not be forced to go to term.

Rheumatoid arthritis usually improves with pregnancy although relapses are not unknown. High doses of steroids to the mother may be responsible for an increased fetal loss and possibly for a raised incidence of congenital abnormality.

(e) SYPHILIS

Pregnancy does not alter the course of the disease in the mother. When syphilis is detected at the first antenatal examination adequate treatment (up to 10 or 12 million units of penicillin at the fifth month) will protect against congenital syphilis in the baby. While not a medical indication for abortion, syphilis may be found in social circumstances where termination is indicated in the case of unwanted pregnancies.

(f) ABDOMINAL EMERGENCIES

The need to terminate a pregnancy may very occasionally arise during the surgical treatment of unrelated conditions and the British 1967 Abortion Act makes provision for this unusual situation (chapter 14). It may be to the patient's advantage, as well as being humane, to terminate pregnancy if extensive malignant disease is found at a laparotomy. Abortion might also be thought necessary in the course of treating a perforated peptic ulcer or bowel in ulcerative colitis, or in the case of acute pancreatitis.[30]

METHODS

All techniques must be preceded by a careful medical and surgical history and a full pelvic examination. The stage of gestation will largely determine the method used and the possibility of the patient deceiving the doctor about the duration of the pregnancy must be borne in mind.

Pregnancy itself usually rules out the possibility of most types of gross pelvic pathology. Intercurrent chest infections should be excluded. When abortion is carried out for social, psychiatric or eugenic reasons it should prove a simple, safe operation, but if the operation is performed on medical grounds the operator may be dealing with someone who is already very ill and the risks will be increased.

The patient should be blood-grouped and a haemoglobin estimation may be indicated. If the patient is anaemic, or any complications are envisaged, blood may be cross matched in advance. Attention should be paid to the possibility of rhesus sensitization following induced abortion.

Abortion in the first trimester, especially when performed by vacuum aspiration, is done as an outpatient procedure in many countries, and in Britain it often involves only one night in hospital. Patients may be admitted on the morning of the operation and discharged late on the next day. If the operation is complicated by infection, signs and symptoms are nearly always apparent within 48 hours.

The operation should only be attempted in a fully equipped operating theatre and the possibility of having to do a laparotomy or even a hysterectomy should be borne in mind.

PROCEDURE

Any suitable general anaesthetic can be used. Ether may cause uterine atony and its use should be avoided if possible. Local anaesthetic can be used for dilatation and curettage and for vacuum aspiration in a small number of multiparous patients coming to termination at less than 12 weeks of pregnancy. Paracervical block using 2 per cent lignocaine has the advantage of relaxing the cervix and may also be used when a general anaesthetic is given. Approximately 3 ml is injected on either side of the cervix in three 1 ml doses at 1, 2 and 4 cm in depth.

Intravenous or intramuscular ergometrine (0·25 mg) can be given before commencing the operation and repeated to a total of 1 mg. Catheterization carries a risk of infection and can be avoided in some operations, although it is dangerous to risk a full bladder when giving a paracervical block.

1   Dilatation and curettage

Full aseptic precautions must be taken and the perineum adequately cleansed. The patient is draped, the vagina swabbed and the pelvis re-examined. It simplifies the operation if a retroverted uterus can be brought into the anteverted position. A speculum is passed and the cervix is gripped with a vosellum or sponge forceps. It is important to make sure the cervix is held securely and to reposition the vosellum if necessary. A sound is passed to confirm the size, position and duration of pregnancy. Dilators are passed gently until Hegar size 12 or 14, taking care not to damage the cervix. Closed sponge or ovum forceps can then be inserted; they are opened inside the uterus, rotated through 90°, closed and withdrawn. The process is repeated until the major part of the products of conception have been removed and the uterus is then curetted. Debris may also be removed with a sterile swab held in sponge forceps. It is important to combine thoroughness with gentleness when curetting the uterus.

Other possible procedures include irrigation with hot saline or antiseptic solution using a flushing curette, but the method may predispose to tubal blockage and has nothing to recommend it.

Bimanual compression of the uterus is useful to stop bleeding.

The dilatation of the cervix with a balloon or using laminaria tents (carefully dried, compressed, sterile sea-tangle) is more gentle than dilatation at operation but carries a risk of infection. On the day preceding the operation the largest tent (or series of tents) that can be passed beyond the internal os is placed in the cervix, under direct vision and with sterile precautions but without anaesthetic. The tent takes up water and swells slowly.

2 Uterine aspiration

The technique of evacuating the uterus using a tube passed through the cervical canal and linked by a flexible connection to some source of suction was introduced by Wu and Wu in 1958.[38] The method has been widely used in Eastern Europe and is now finding favour in Western practice. It has been fully reviewed by Kerslake and Casey.[39]

Metal or plastic suction curettes can be used. With the former the internal diameter in millimeters should be equal to the length of gestation in weeks, but plastic curettes have thicker walls and consequently a larger external diameter. Plastic curettes are also more difficult to sterilize but they enable the operator to observe the passage of the products of conception very easily and may be more gentle on the uterus. A variety of curette endings has been devised with the mouth placed terminally or at the side. The opportunity to control the duration and amount of suction by a thumb-controlled air hole in the stem is an advantage. The curette is joined to the suction apparatus by a flexible rubber or polyethylene pressure tube, and when an opaque curette is used a glass or plastic union is included in the suction so that the passage of the products of conception can be observed. The suction tube is connected via a glass settling bottle. A pressure of 300 mm mercury or below is used and any adequate suction pump can be employed (figure 35). A theatre surgical suction pump is sometimes used but it is important to have a foolproof

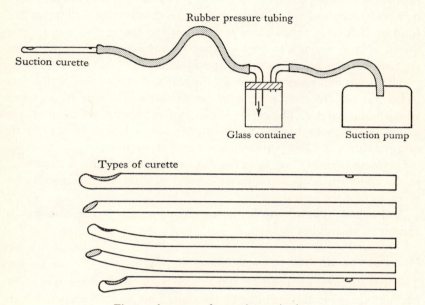

Fig. 35. Apparatus for uterine aspiration.

system for ensuring that under no circumstances can air be blown out of the curette. It should be routine to test that the curette is sucking by placing the mouth against a sterile glove or towel. A modification for developing countries has been to use a vacuum bottle which is evacuated either by pumping or by burning alcohol in it before the operation is carried out.[40]

3 Hysterotomy

Hysterotomy is often regarded as the method of choice for performing an abortion after the twelfth to fourteenth week of pregnancy. Haemorrhage can be controlled and there should be little risk of infection.

A woman having a hysterotomy should be warned that she should have any future deliveries in hospital.

(a) ABDOMINAL HYSTEROTOMY

The operation is usually performed under a general anaesthetic although spinal anaesthesia is possible. Access is most suitably obtained through a transverse, phannensteil incision which leaves the least visible scar. If the operation is to be combined with tubal ligation, the uterus is opened by a short longitudinal mid-line incision of the anterior wall below the fundus. If further pregnancies may follow the hysterotomy and if the uterus is large enough to have a defined lower segment, a small lower segment caesarean section may be performed.

The ovum will protrude through the scar and can be delivered intact in many cases. In early pregnancy the thick decidua may be removed with a blunt curette. The cervix is dilated from above and the uterus is closed in one or two layers using interrupted or herringbone chromic catgut sutures and the peritoneum sutured separately.[41]

Oxytocin (5 units) may be given directly into the uterine wall as soon as the abdomen is open and intramuscular or intravenous ergot can be given during the operation.

Abdominal hysterotomy is the logical operation if late abortion is combined with tubal ligation.

(b) VAGINAL HYSTEROTOMY

The uterine supports must be sufficiently lax to allow the cervix to be brought almost to the introitus by traction. This limits the operation to multiparous patients under 16 weeks of pregnancy and even in this group the procedure has no real advantages over the abdominal approach and the disadvantage of providing poor access and making it more difficult to deal with emergencies. Tubal ligation combined with vaginal hysterotomy has a significant failure rate.

The operation can be carried out under general or local anaesthetic (40 ml 0·5 per cent lignocaine). The perineum is cleansed, the bladder catheterized, the patient draped, a speculum passed and the cervix is held and brought to the lower end of the vagina. Ergometrine (0·5 mg) can be injected into the uterine wall. The cervix is dilated as far as possible without damage and an incision is made in the upper 4 to 5 cm of the vaginal wall, the bladder is separated from the uterus and retracted and the dissection is continued until the peritoneum is reached.

A longitudinal incision is then made in the anterior wall of the cervix, the fetal membranes will bulge out of the incision and the products of conception are removed with ovum forceps.

The uterine cavity is curetted and the cervical incision repaired with two layers of catgut sutures. The vagina wall is repaired separately.

4   Intra-amniotic injections

In the 1930s it was noticed that the injection of radio-opaque media for amniography often induced premature labour and in 1934 Aburel[42] used intra-amniotic injections to terminate early pregnancy. In the past few years there has been renewed interest in the use of hypertonic solutions to induce abortion and the method is a useful one in the second trimester of pregnancy although it involves certain dangers and must be used with care.

The uterus can be approached through the vagina or (after 16 weeks) the abdominal wall. Full sterile precautions must be taken and the operation performed in an operating theatre. When the abdominal route is chosen a 17-gauge spinal anaesthetic needle and stylet or a size 14 trocar and cannula with a 2 mm (external diameter) polyethylene catheter are used. The latter is less likely to become displaced during the procedure. Following local anaesthesia, the needle is introduced below the umbilicus and slightly to the right or left away from the fetal back. Care must be taken to avoid the bladder, which should be empty. Amniocentesis is performed and 200 ml of liquor aspirated and replaced by an equal volume of 20 per cent saline or 50 per cent glucose. A reservoir and two-way tap system can be used. The injection must be made slowly, great care must be taken to ensure that the needle is not in the intervellous space or in a blood vessel and the patient should be observed closely and the injection stopped if she complains of pain or untoward symptoms. For these reasons, and because of the intrinsic risks, general anaesthesia should be avoided. As a prophylactic measure 0·5 gm of oxytetracycline can be added to the replacement fluid. Labour generally follows within one to two days but may sometimes be delayed for a further 24 hours. The conceptus is normally expelled cleanly and curettage is rarely necessary. In late pregnancy, induction of labour can be supplemented by an oxytocin drip.

The action of hypertonic solutions in inducing abortion is not fully understood. It seems unlikely that it is a simple mechanical response to uterine distension. The injected solution damages the placenta and may have a local effect on the uterine wall. In rabbits the effect can be antagonized by giving progesterone.

The method is contra-indicated for therapeutic termination in cases of cardiac or renal disease or toxaemia, because the sodium concentration serum volume and osmolarity will rise.

The risks of amniotic-fluid replacement are intrauterine infection, the possibility of injection into the placental intervellous space and the danger of brain damage. Glucose may predispose to infection more than saline but staphylococci can survive even in 25 per cent saline. Deaths due to pontine and basal ganglia infarction following within a few hours of amniotic-fluid replacement have been reported.[43] The cerebral damage probably resulted from excessive dehydration but the possibility of intravenous injection cannot be excluded. Wagatsuma[44] has reported on 25 deaths following the use of intra-amniotic hypertonic saline solutions.

5   Abortifacient paste

Medicated soaps are available for intrauterine injection. Using full sterile precautions, and if necessary with a general anaesthetic, a sterile cannula, about the size of an IUD introducer, is passed along the cervical canal and 10 to 30 ml (depending upon the duration of the pregnancy) of paste is introduced into the uterine lumen. Abortion usually occurs within 20 to 30 hours, but curettage may be necessary later.

No objective evaluation of the method has been attempted. The method was introduced in Germany and twenty-five fatalities were reported in the literature of the 1930s. There is a risk of infection, haemorrhage during the abortion, haemolysis and pulmonary embolism.[45] The paste appears to spread over a large area of the uterine wall. The method has no advantage over vacuum aspiration or dilatation and curettage during the first three months of pregnancy, but it may present a reasonable alternative to hysterotomy in selected cases between three and five months of pregnancy and it has the advantage of not damaging the cervix.

6   Abortifacient drugs

Very little research has been done on abortifacient drugs, although there can be little doubt that they would be widely used if developed. Possible lines of research are discussed in chapter 16.

Oestrogens, quinine and oxytocin have all proved unreliable as a method of inducing abortion in early pregnancy. Very small-scale clinical trials of aminopterin (4-aminopteroylglutamic acid) have been carried out.[46] Like most possible abortifacients it is also teratogenic and it is likely that any drug which was used on a wide scale would have to be backed by the possibility of surgically induced abortion if it failed.

SIDE EFFECTS

1 Medical and surgical

Two facts of cardinal importance must be kept in mind when considering the complications of induced abortion. First, for each specific method the risks of the operation rise sharply with increasing duration of pregnancy, and in practice the gulf is widened by the fact that before the twelfth week dilatation and curettage and vacuum aspiration account for nearly all cases, while after this time vaginal and abdominal hysterotomy make up the majority of operations. Secondly, as in all surgical procedures, the operator must perform terminations reasonably often in order to be fully competent.

In assessing the risks of termination it should be noted that the danger is usually increased in those women where, for medical or obstetric reasons, pregnancy also carried unusual risks. It is also important to remember that a significant number of women refused legal abortions turn to backstreet abortionists. Over half the patients admitted with criminal abortions in New York hospitals were febrile and 1 in 20 critically ill.

In recent years a revolution has occurred in the safety of legal abortion. Death rates have fallen in all the large published series, especially in those countries where abortion is available on social as well as medical grounds. The low mortality and morbidity rates quoted for some Eastern European countries have been called 'unreliable, vague and in some cases utopian'. Whilst it is true that the reliability of vital statistics from different countries varies, there is evidence that in Czechoslovakia, Hungary and Northern Yugoslavia impeccable records are kept and adequate follow-up carried out. The compact nature of the countries, the high incidence of hospital care and the excellent standard of medicine (the maternal mortality rates in Czechoslovakia and England were exactly the same in 1962) make their statistics particularly trustworthy.

(a) INFLAMMATION AND OTHER IMMEDIATE COMPLICATIONS

It is unreasonable to suppose that an operation of the relative simplicity of abortion, open to the limited number of permutations of procedure that are possible, gives rise to the range and incidence of complications that is sometimes quoted. For example, Mehlan[47] quotes a rate of 0·8 per cent and Topp[48] 55·60 per cent for inflammation. It must be assumed that authors are confused by the unavoidable difficulties of categorizing non-lethal symptoms, by variations in the length and diligence of follow-up and by an unscientific desire to justify preconceived notions of the excessive dangers (or safety) of induced abortion. Undoubtedly, the incidence of serious complications lies closer to the 1 per cent range than the 50 per cent. Mehlan's statistics have the virtue of being based on a large series (145,000). Vacuum aspiration probably leads to fewest inflammatory complications (0·8 to 5 per cent).[39]

Černoch[49] quotes an incidence of 5 per cent immediate complication in dilatation and curettage. Lindahl[50] records serious complications in 36 of 983 (3·7 per cent) women having vaginal hysterotomies and in the Danish series of 5,320 abdominal hysterotomies there were 113 (2·1 per cent) non-fatal, serious complications.[51] The majority of published series fit into the 2 to 5 per cent range for immediate complications (see Lindahl for discussion). Perhaps the most objective measure of short-term operative complications is the number of women who have to be readmitted to hospital within four weeks of a legal abortion. In Hungary (1964) 0·47 per cent were readmitted because of fever and 1·02 per cent because of haemorrhage; and immediate complications (perforation, haemorrhage, fever) recorded at the time of the operation were 1·12 per cent.[6]

The number of previous children and induced abortions has not been demonstrated to have an influence on the incidence of complications but the risks of termination are greater in the very young (under 17 years old). However, the hazards of birth are also raised in the very young in whom toxaemia is common, eclampsia can follow suddenly and the caesarean section and perinatal mortality rates are increased.

(b) HAEMORRHAGE

Vacuum aspiration before twelve weeks is associated with least loss. In comparable series Vladov et al.[52] found an average loss of 66 ml with vacuum aspiration and 85 ml with dilatation and curettage. Between 1 and 2 per cent of patients having legal abortions early in pregnancy in Hungary are registered as having haemorrhages as a result of the operation. The blood loss rises with the length of gestation, whatever method of termination is used. In Sweden the law is slow and cumbersome, and in a series of over 1,000 induced abortions a mere 5 per cent were terminated before the twelfth week and over half after the seventeenth week, but nevertheless only 32 cases of major haemorrhage occurred during the operation, of which five required intravenous replacement therapy.[50]

(c) PERFORATION

The incidence of perforation in dilatation and curettage operations has been put at between 0·09 and 6 per cent.[39] The wide differences are once again largely due to differences in legal and obstetric practice, although some cases of perforation may go undiagnosed. Perforations with vacuum aspiration are certainly less than 1 in 1,000 and may be less than in 1 10,000.

If it is thought that the uterus has been perforated, and that either bowel or omentum has been damaged at the time of perforation, then a laparotomy should be performed immediately rather than instituting conservative measures until symptoms appear.

(d) DEATH

The mortality rate for legal abortion varies in different countries (table 20). It is related to the law and medical practice of the nations concerned being highest in Sweden and lowest in Czechoslovakia and Hungary.

TABLE 20. *Mortality from legal abortion*

Country	Number of abortions	Deaths	Deaths/1,000 operations
Japan (1954)	108,055	8	0·08
Yugoslavia (1960–1)	177,499	8	0·04
Czechoslovakia (1958–64)	561,000	12	0·02
Hungary (1963–4)	328,200	2	0·006

Deaths from pregnancy and childbirth (all causes).
United Kingdom (1964) 0·2 per 1,000 deliveries.

The trained physician who works outside the law in countries where there are strict anti-abortion laws can also achieve a very low mortality rate. Timanus had two deaths in 5,210 criminal abortions in Maryland (0·4/1,000) and others have an even better record.[53]

A disproportionate number of fatalities occurs to women who are being terminated on medical and not on social or eugenic grounds. In Lindahl's follow-up of 1,000 cases in Sweden the only death was one multiparous woman having a vaginal hysterotomy and sterilization for chronic nephritis performed when she was 17 to 20 weeks pregnant. The highest mortality for hospital abortions in recent times was that of Winter's[54] series where there were thirteen deaths among 574 cases (2·3 per cent), but the operations were for medical indications and a significant proportion after the fourth month.

Today, when the abortion is performed early in gestation by an experienced operator, and when it is done for social, psychiatric or medical indications, there can be no doubt that it involves less risk to life than carrying the pregnancy to term.

(e) STERILITY

Among remote complications of abortion sterility is probably the most important. Menstrual patterns are found to be unchanged in over 95 per cent of patients after vacuum aspiration and no change in ovarian anatomy or in the incidence of anovulatory cycles is found after other methods of termination. The most thorough long-term follow-up of patients has been Lindahl's[50] of 1,132 legal abortions in Sweden: in the first three weeks after the operation sixteen women presented with salpingitis and thirteen with endometritis, but when the same group of patients was followed up one to five years later 1·6 per cent showed tubal abnormalities which might have been due to the preceding abortion. In a number of patients tubal changes were attributed to episodes of salpingitis which preceded the legal abortion and there was little correlation between the immediate post-operative course and subsequent findings. One hundred and sixty-eight women had intrauterine pregnancies after the termination, five complained of involuntary infertility and in one case this was thought to be a consequence of legal abortion.

When reviewing the risk of sterility for an individual woman it must be remembered that the majority of women having terminations already have a family and are seeking an abortion because they do not want any more children, and many women refused legal abortions seek backstreet abortions where there is a much higher risk of complications.

(f) RISKS TO SUBSEQUENT PREGNANCIES

In Hungary, the prematurity rate has risen in recent years and is now the highest in Europe. It is 11 to 12 per cent overall rising to 15 per cent in the towns. It is widely felt that this change is the result of the free recourse to abortion possible in Hungary and particularly to the termination of first pregnancies (table 21).

TABLE 21. *Prematurity and legal abortion (Hungary)*

Previous induced abortions	Prematurity rate (%) (under 2,500 g)
0	10·1
1	14·4
2	16·0
3+	20·5

No change in the incidence of spontaneous abortions and premature deliveries has been discovered after hysterotomy.

No relationship has been found between ectopic pregnancy and previous abortion.

(g) ENDOMETRIOSIS

Endometriosis has been reported in up to 20 per cent of patients one to four years after hysterotomy. It becomes more common with the passage of time since the hysterotomy, and some series may underestimate this complication. In approximately 1 per cent of patients the endometriosis involves the bladder. Fortunately, the lesions are almost always symptomless.[50]

A raised incidence of endometriosis has not been reported after dilatation and curettage or vacuum aspiration.

(h) RHESUS SENSITIZATION

Surgical termination of pregnancy is associated with an increased number of fetal erythrocytes in the maternal circulation.[55] It is not known if sensitization can occur at this time or if any particular method is more or less dangerous and long-term follow-up of this possibility is needed, especially as prophylactic measures might be taken using anti-D immunoglobin.

2 Psychological

The foundations of a woman's psychological and emotional response to termination are laid on the first occasion she seeks advice from a doctor and are built up by all those in whose care she subsequently finds herself. If she is made to feel guilty and if the termination is openly regarded by all around her as disgusting and hateful then many women will feel remorse. For example, the proposition that 'a woman is a uterus surrounded by a supporting organism and directing personality' (Gladstone) is not likely to provide a guilt-free atmosphere in which to have a pregnancy terminated. In a wide review of the literature dealing with the psychiatric sequelae of abortion Simon and Senturia[56] found the incidence of severe guilt variously reported as between zero and 43 per cent. No doubt the variety of background attitudes in which a patient found herself, as well as differing moral and religious drives among the observers, account for this range of differences.

Immediate guilt is rare, and[57, 58] long-term reactions are difficult to assess. Induced abortion and depression are sufficiently common for both to occur in a large number of individuals. There is a low incidence of psychiatric ill effects from induced abortion and in Gebhard's[5] series only 4·2 per cent of the women who had had illegal abortions reported on unfavourable psychiatric consequences. In spite of the worry, pain and degradation that may go with criminal abortion it is excessively rare to find it a precipitating factor in psychiatric illness.

Legal abortion can affect a woman's attitude towards her sexual life, about a quarter feeling it is less satisfactory, an equal number improved and the remainder unchanged. However, any pregnancy, whatever its outcome, alters a woman's attitude to intercourse, and a term delivery worsens subsequent sexual relations in a higher percentage of women than a termination.[59]

3 Social

Most induced abortions are carried out for social reasons; therefore the social consequences of the operation must be considered.

The total number of abortions taking place in a community is probably not greatly affected by the law relating to abortion. When termination is permitted on social grounds numerous abortions are transferred from the criminal section to hospitals. In 1952, in Hungary there were 185,000 live births and 1,700 legal abortions; the law was altered in 1956 and by 1964 there were 184,000 in one year. However, the number of live births in 1964 was 132,100 (figure 36). Therefore the great majority of the legal abortions taking place must have previously occurred illegally. It might be argued that the complete freedom of the Hungarian law (it is impossible for a doctor to refuse a woman an abortion in the first three months of pregnancy) has led to some overall increase in the number of abortions taking place, but it is notable that the birth rate was falling before the law relating to abortion was altered and it may be that, in the presence of rather poor contraceptive services, the number of abortions would have risen anyway.

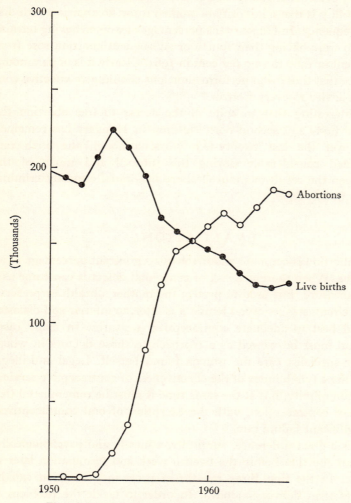

Fig. 36. Live births and legal abortions in Hungary, 1950–65.

Deaths from criminal abortion provide some yardstick of the number taking place and in Hungary, Poland and Czechoslovakia these have fallen by two-thirds or more since the introduction of legislation permitting abortion on social grounds. The decline is greater than that which has taken place in other countries as the result of improved gynaecological care.[6]

The only evidence that legalized abortion may cause any kind of social irresponsibility is that a minority of women resort to abortion with distressing frequency. In Hungary the percentage of women having terminations who were having their fourth or subsequent abortion rose from 11·9 per cent in 1960 to 15·9 per cent in 1964. Clearly it is of paramount importance that those who perform abortions should give effective contraceptive advice to every woman.

It is interesting that in spite of the access to free abortion the number of first- and second-born children in Hungary has remained constant over the last twenty-five years, although the birth rate has declined considerably during this interval and much of the fall has been the result of induced abortion—initially mostly criminal and lately mostly legal.

EVALUATION

Induced abortion is common and involves a significant percentage of all conceptions. When there is a risk of congenital defect it can come as a welcome measure. But used to protect the mother's health or preserve the social circumstances of her family it is often an inferior and distasteful second best to adequate contraceptive measures. In many cases termination must be viewed as a reproach to those doctors in whose general or specialist care the woman found herself. Legal and illegal abortions are a rough index of the effectiveness of contraceptive services within a community, but at the same time it must be remembered that all forms of contraception, with the exception of oral contraceptives, have a significant failure rate.

There is a great difference, surgically, ethically and psychologically, between an abortion before the twelfth week and termination later in pregnancy. In the first three months of pregnancy abortion can be made safer than delivery at term. In order to tackle the problem of criminal abortion realistically it may be wise to interpret the indications for termination widely in the first trimester, but it is probably in the woman's best interests to err on the side of strictness after twelve weeks.

Vacuum aspiration is the safest method of termination in the first three months of pregnancy, but in the hands of the experienced surgeon dilatation and curettage is also a satisfactory operation. In those circumstances when abortion has to be done after the twelfth to fourteenth week abdominal hysterotomy is the method of choice.

Every woman who has an induced abortion must be offered appropriate contraceptive advice. Oral contraception can be begun five days after a termination or an IUD can be inserted at the time of operation.

14 LEGAL AND ADMINISTRATIVE ASPECTS OF BIRTH CONTROL

In most countries of the world contemporary statute law represents the prevailing social values of earlier generations; in others it embodies the ideologies or aspiration of a ruling group; in only a few does it attempt to cope with the realities of existing social and economic conditions. In relation to the control of conception the countries of Western Europe and North America fall broadly into the first category, the communist countries of Eastern Europe and of Asia belong to the second whilst a number of developing societies, amongst them Japan and India, may be regarded as members of the third, although there are unexpected deficiencies in their legislation; in India, for example, there has been no reform of the law on abortion.

The law, in the majority of Western countries, has reflected the doctrine of the mediaeval church in regarding procreation as the primary purpose of marriage. This is especially true of Roman Catholic countries in Europe, but even in England and the United States a similar outlook has, until recently, prevailed: all attempts to frustrate the process of parenthood have been discouraged by the government and by the courts. The ideological orientation of communist states is fundamentally pronatalist, the advocacy of family limitation on economic grounds being contrary to Marxist doctrine; in recent years, however, there has been a greater awareness of the value of birth control in promoting maternal and infant health. It is only in a small, though growing, number of countries that family limitation is positively encouraged by governments through programmes which have included legalized abortion as well as contraception and sterilization.

Doctors practising in the field of contraception may find themselves working in an area where the law is unclear or possibly even hostile. The doctor is responsible for being well informed on the law and in the United States he must also be familiar with the legislation of his own particular state. Accurate, detailed clinical records should be kept, especially in the case of sterilization and therapeutic termination.

CONTRACEPTION AND THE LAW

1   England

There are, in England, no legal restrictions on the use of contraceptives or on the publication of birth control information provided this does not contravene the requirements of the Obscene Publications Act of 1857 under which the early birth control propagandists were prosecuted. Nor has the manufacture and sale of contraceptives ever been forbidden by English law, and existing legal restrictions are few and trivial. The sale of contraceptives through vending machines in public places is prohibited by most local authorities by virtue of their having adopted a model by-law circulated by the Home Office in 1949. Section 4 (5) of the 1954 Television Act[1] precludes the advertising on television of 'contraceptives, matrimonial agencies, fortune tellers and undertakers'. Other public authorities, notably the London Passenger Transport Board, have arbitrarily refused advertisements by the Family Planning Association on the grounds that these 'might give offence to minorities'.

The major legislative issue, in relation to birth control, in England has been the extent to which local authorities and doctors working in the National Health Service should be allowed to provide contraception as a charge against public funds. A basic aim of the early birth control movement was to persuade the government to extend its maternal and child welfare functions to the giving of contraceptive information. Partial success was achieved in 1930 when the Ministry of Health, through its Memorandum 153 MCW, permitted existing Child Welfare Centres to give contraceptive advice 'to married women for whom a further pregnancy would be detrimental to health'. This instruction was liberally interpreted by most local authorities and the history of the English birth control movement after 1930 is a record of increasing local authority subsidization of the voluntary clinics through the provision of rent-free premises and financial grants.[2]

The 1949 *Report* of the Royal Commission on Population recommended that contraceptive advice should be available to all women who require it and that the initial duty to give this advice should rest with the family doctor. It was only after the introduction of the Pill, in the early 1960s, that general practitioners became extensively involved in family planning and the distinction between 'medical' and 'other' grounds was carried over into surgery practice. The Ministry's ruling is that doctors may provide free advice to any woman who requests it but that free contraceptive supplies may only be prescribed for those who require them on 'medical' grounds; for 'social' cases a charge must be made.

The Family Planning Act of 1967 removes this somewhat tenuous distinction but only in the field of local authority provision; in the hospital service and in general practice it remains, though it will become meaningless with the abolition of the tripartite system, as envisaged in the Minister's Green Paper.[3] The Act has two further implications for the future of birth control provision in England. By deliberately avoiding the term 'married women' which appeared in the 1930 Memorandum it encourages local authorities to take a permissive attitude on the much-discussed question of providing contraceptive advice to single women. And by giving the Minister powers to ensure that acceptable standards are reached in all areas it enables Members of Parliament to draw attention to those authorities which fail to take advantage of its provisions.

The 1967 Act was the outcome of many years of sustained pressure on the British government to extend the provisions of the 1930 Memorandum; the campaign culminated in a private members' bill which, in the event, was facilitated by the government. Although the need for the extension of domiciliary birth control services was frequently mentioned in the parliamentary debates on the Family Planning Bill, authority to operate such schemes derives from the 1963 Children's and Young Persons' Act which places on local authorities the responsibility for providing services to families which may prevent children being taken into care or before the courts.

There are several ways in which the quality and harmlessness of contraceptive products are regulated by law. As with other pharmaceutical preparations the active ingredients in chemical spermicides must be disclosed on the package and the use of the BSI 'Kitemark' ensures that condoms reach a certain standard of quality. In English law oral contraceptives come under Schedule 4 of the Poisons Act and all supplies must carry the designation and address of the supplier. Since 1964 the Committee on the Safety of Drugs (Dunlop Committee) has scrutinized all new oral preparations and has alerted doctors to the need for systematic reporting of side effects.

2 The United States

In America the sale and distribution of contraceptives is governed by both federal and, in some cases, state laws. The relevant federal statute is the notorious Comstock Act of 1873 which declares contraceptives obscene and prohibits their transmission through the mails or by public carriers. The ban also covers literature which either describes birth control methods or advises where they may be obtained. Although rigidly enforced until 1930, since that date the effectiveness of the Act has been eroded by judicial interpretation. A major breach in the statute was made in 1936 in the course of a prosecution of a doctor who had imported from Japan a supply of diaphragms which were seized by the customs. The case, which became known as 'The United States *vs* One Package', went to appeal where Justice Augustus Hand exempted from Comstock and related Acts 'the importation, sale or carriage by mail of things which might intelligently be employed by conscientious and competent physicians for the purpose of saving life or promoting the well-being of their patients'.

The courts will now exempt from the provisions of the Comstock Act all activities of reputable manufacturers and members of the medical profession and the Planned Parenthood League no longer takes the precaution of consigning contraceptives or birth control literature under a doctor's signature since the Federal Court overruled the decision of the state legislature in the case of Griswald v. Connecticut.

State laws, where they exist, have similarly been modified by judicial interpretations and, exceptionally, by subsequent amendment of the relevant statute. There are at present thirty states which have laws affecting birth control. In seventeen there is a prohibition of all activities connected with contraception but doctors and other qualified persons are specifically exempted from their provisions, birth control clinics operate freely and contraceptives are openly sold at drugstores. In eight other states the only legal obstacle is a ban on contraceptive advertising and in the remaining five states which ban all sales of contraceptives the law does not interfere with bona fide medical practice.

The Planned Parenthood League (now Planned Parenthood–World Population) operates birth control clinics in all states and voluntary effort is now being reinforced by federal and state provision. The change in official attitudes followed President Johnson's health and education message to Congress in 1966 in which he declared: 'It is essential that all families have access to information and services that will allow freedom to choose the number and spacing of their children within the dictates of individual conscience'. In 1968 Congress was persuaded to earmark 6 per cent of the health, education and welfare budget ($24 millions) for family planning services and state legislatures quickly followed the federal lead.[4] Between 1960 and 1967 the number of states whose health departments provided contraceptive services increased from 7 to 37 and 23 per cent of 'medically indigent' women now obtain family planning aid from voluntary clinics, state health departments or hospitals or from private doctors acting under the Social Security Act (Title XIX).

The American Food and Drug Administration is given the responsibility of controlling the quality of all condoms and diaphragms which form the basis of interstate traffic; violations of the requirements of the FDA Act (see chapter 3) may attract penalties of three years imprisonment or fines of $10,000. An additional discipline which applies to offending manufacturers in the US (but not in Britain) is that test results are published.

The federal government also controls the sale of drugs in the United States under the Food, Drug and Cosmetic Act passed in 1906. This was revised in 1938 after more than one hundred people died from taking sulfanilamide diluted in ethylene glycol (an untested solvent) and again in 1962 in the light of the European thalidomide tragedy. All oral contraceptives must meet the requirements of the Act and the Food and Drug Administration established one of the first committees, in 1963, for the large-scale investigation of thrombo-embolic phenomena. The Food and Drug Administration can oblige manufacturers to print any dangers associated with a preparation on the packet and this has now been done in the case of thrombo-embolic phenomena and oral contraceptives.

3 Other Countries

In the rest of the world official attitudes to contraception vary all the way from outright condemnation to government participation and provision. In France the legal status of contraception, under a law of 1920, approximated to the situation in Connecticut until the concessions made in 1968. At the other extreme, Danish law *requires* a doctor attending a woman who has a term delivery or an abortion to offer contraceptive advice. Though, in practice it is unlikely that action would ever be taken against a medical practitioner who failed to offer such help (and the statute may to this extent be regarded merely as the expression of a pious aspiration), its existence nevertheless represents a civilized ideal and it has not been found to cause offence to women. In Poland a similar law requires a practitioner to give contraceptive advice after terminating a pregnancy. Attitudes of this type are in vivid contrast to the frivolous stance adopted by many doctors and nurses in other Western countries who have been known to wave goodbye to the newly delivered mother from the door of the maternity home saying: 'See you next year, dear.'

Most Scandinavian countries have well-developed clinic services and attempts are now being made to popularize contraception in the Soviet Union and the East European countries. In Germany birth control is not encouraged; in Spain and Portugal it is not mentioned. Government intervention in favour of birth control is most frequent in Asia and is least developed in Latin America.

4 Contraception and the Patent Law

There are important patent rights controlling the sale and distribution of IUDs. Plastic devices cost two to three cents in materials and production; they sell at between ten and one hundred times this price. Different patents have been taken out for open-ended devices, for double coils, for introducers and for the idea of using the strings to draw the device into the introducer. Rights usually extend to all countries in the world, although sometimes they have been partly relaxed in a limited number of developing nations.

It is unfortunate that Patent Officers have allowed applications for such simple and self-evident devices which have a long history, require little or no research and investment, and which are particularly suitable for poor women. Anyone who believes he can advance contraceptive technology should take advice from one of the world family planning organizations to ensure that the ethically unassailable tradition of making medical procedures freely available to those that need them are preserved: contraceptives, like penicillin, should not be patented, although certain steps may be commercially necessary when oral contraceptives, demanding a sophisticated technology and large capital investment, are produced.

VOLUNTARY STERILIZATION
1 England

In the absence of either legislation or case law the status of voluntary sterilization in England is a matter of uncertainty and speculation. The 1934 Brock Committee's recommendations that voluntary sterilization should, for certain specified reasons, be made legal were never implemented and the indications proposed at that date, being concerned with eugenic rather than socio-economic indications, have since been overtaken by changing social needs. In the face of conflicting interpretations of the laws which have from time to time been suggested, the medical defence societies of England and Scotland simultaneously sought counsel's opinions in 1960.[5]

The English counsel's opinion was that an operation for sterilization is not unlawful whether it is performed on therapeutic or eugenic grounds or for any other reasons, provided that there is full and valid consent to the operation by the patient concerned. Counsel pointed out that the proposition, never having been tested in the courts, had no direct judicial support and that a test case would establish a precedent of the utmost significance. Although convinced that the courts would uphold the legality of such an operation on therapeutic or well-founded eugenic grounds, counsel stressed that the risk of an adverse finding would increase as the reasons for the operation became less well founded.

Scottish counsel expressed the opinion that if such an operation were performed by a responsible surgeon, with the full consent of the patient and if the reason for doing it was substantial and not obviously immoral by present-day standards, it would be exceedingly improbable that a court would regard the act as criminal. Commenting on these statements, the *British Medical Journal* concluded: 'Whatever may be the law on sterilization, it is clearly most desirable that the courts or Parliament should now declare it.'[5] The Medical Defence Union has laid down certain safeguards and has issued a form of consent requiring the signatures of both spouses before the operation is conducted. The Union has stated that in the event of a doctor becoming involved in litigation it would fully support him.

2 The United States

There is no federal law dealing with voluntary sterilization in America, and in most states the same ambiguity exists as in England. Legal counsel have ruled that 'there can be no question as to the legality of sterilization performed upon the basis of therapeutic indications. Such sterilization need not be performed to save the patient's life; it is sufficient that such an operation will, in the opinion of the attending physician, be for the protection and in the best interests of the patient's well-being'. Connecticut and Utah are exceptions, having statutes specifically requiring medical necessity. In a number of other states the law has been amended to the more liberal interpretation.

3 Other Countries

Apart from such countries as India and Puerto Rico where sterilization is actively encouraged by government, the law in most countries is either unresolved as in Britain or sterilization is limited to eugenic abnormalities. Swedish legislation is notable in allowing sterilization on eugenic, medical and social grounds; a similar law operates in Denmark.

ABORTION LAW

1 England

Before April 1968, when the 1967 Abortion Act became operative, the legality of medical termination of pregnancy in England rested on a hopeful interpretation of case law which was by no means universally accepted by academic lawyers.[6] The basic statute was the Offences Against the Persons Act of 1861 which made abortion, in any circumstances, an offence attracting a maximum penalty of penal servitude for life. The precedent, exempting from the provisions of the Act cases in which termination was carried out in order to save or preserve the woman's life, was the Bourne judgement of 1938, in which a London gynaecologist was acquitted after terminating a 14-year-old girl. The girl had been raped by soldiers and the special circumstances of the case were held to constitute a slender precedent.

The 1967 Act not only codifies what previously rested on case law; for the first time, it legalizes abortion on grounds other than the preservation of the woman's life. The Act states that a doctor may terminate a pregnancy if he and another doctor consider:

'(a) that the continuance of the pregnancy would involve risk to the life of the pregnant woman or if injury to the physical or mental health of the pregnant woman or any existing children of her family greater than if the pregnancy were terminated; or
(b) that there is a substantial risk that if the child were born it would suffer from such physical or mental abnormalities as to be seriously handicapped.'

The Act directs that, in balancing the relative risks of pregnancy and termination under (a), account may be taken of the 'woman's actual or reasonably foreseeable environment', and it requires that the termination be carried out in an approved hospital except in cases of 'immediate necessity' when the need for a second opinion is also dispensed with. Legal and medical comment on the 1967 Act has been provided by a number of interested bodies.

2 The United States

Until 1967 only four states permitted abortion on grounds other than to preserve the life of the mother. Colorado, New Mexico, Alabama and the District of Columbia allowed termination to prevent 'serious and permanent bodily injury' or to protect the health of the mother. The United States' laws are particularly restrictive because the burden of proving 'necessity' is invariably assumed to lie with the defendant, and doctors have been reluctant to operate in any case which might be challenged.[7]

The term 'therapeutic abortion' in the US has not been extended, as in most other countries, to cover abortion on psychiatric or even eugenic grounds. Thus, though there is evidence that rubella contracted before the twelfth week of pregnancy produces congenital abnormality in 30 per cent of cases, the mother's life is not in danger, abortion would be clearly illegal and, consequently, doctors rarely intervene. Indeed, whereas in most countries there has been a rise in the number of therapeutic abortions during the last 20 years, in the US there has been a decline, despite the fact that reporting is assumed to be better than formerly.[8]

Very recently the situation has changed rapidly. In 1967 abortion law reform bills were introduced into thirty state legislatures and in five states the statutes have already been amended.

Most attempts to alter state law revolve around the American Law Institute Model Penal Code (§ 250.3) which permits termination by a licensed physician if he believes (a) the continuation of the pregnancy would gravely impair the physical or mental health of the mother; (b) the child would be born with a grave physical or mental defect; or (c) the pregnancy resulted from rape, incest or felonious intercourse.

Surveys among American obstetricians show that the majority approve of the Model Penal Code proposals.[9]

3 Other Countries

In the majority of countries of the world abortion is illegal and if an exception is made to allow a doctor, acting in good faith and on grounds of medical necessity, to operate his right to do so is more often tacitly conceded than statutorily assured. The pressure for abortion law reform is increasing in many parts of the world and much attention is being paid to the experiences of the dozen or so countries which have liberalized their laws. One of the first countries in the world to do so was the Soviet Union which, in 1920, revised its statutes to allow abortion at the request of the pregnant woman.

Statutes dealing with abortion were passed by a number of Scandinavian countries during the 1930s: in Iceland in 1935, in Sweden in 1938 and in Denmark in 1939. Some of these laws were rather restrictive and subsequent revisions were made to include social, economic and ethical considerations. Especially in Sweden, where even after the changes enacted in 1946 legislation still proved unsatisfactory, and in Denmark, where the delay necessitated by tribunal procedure is reflected in unnecessarily high mortality rates (see p. 203), there is dissatisfaction with existing laws. The Nordic Council is at present examining the legislation of all Scandinavian countries and it is expected that more liberal statutes will be enacted. In 1947 the German Democratic Republic legislated to permit abortion for a range of medical and social indications and though there was, between 1950 and 1965, a reversion to the strictly medical interpretation, the broader grounds, including specific consideration of the woman's environment, were reinstated in March 1965.

Outside Europe a country whose policies have been much discussed is Japan where, in 1948, abortion was made universally available in an attempt to control population growth. In this respect the policy was successful and total abortions reached a peak of 1,159,288 in 1956, a year in which total live births numbered 1,665,278; since that year, largely due to a policy of contraceptive provision, the number of legal abortions has dropped to approximately three-quarters of a million per year.

The other major group of countries which have legalized abortion on non-medical grounds are the socialist countries of Eastern Europe—Czechoslovakia, Bulgaria, Hungary, Poland, Rumania and Yugoslavia —where, between 1956 and 1960, laws were enacted to allow termination for economic and social, as well as medical, indications. The conditions under which termination may be obtained are not, of course, identical in each of the six countries. In Czechoslovakia, for example, the qualifying grounds are catalogued in a supplementary decree, but in Hungary and Rumania abortion must be granted if the woman insists. In all countries where there has been a liberalization of the law there has been an immediate increase in the number of therapeutic abortions, but the extent of criminal abortion has subsequently declined. With the development of effective contraceptive services the trend noted in Japan may prove to be universal for countries where abortion is legalized.

MEDICAL ETHICS

Most physicians try to follow a particular pattern of medical ethics and, in the controversial field of contraception and abortion, their sincere convictions may come into conflict with statute law. Only very rarely will a doctor feel obliged to carry out a procedure which society regards as criminal. More commonly, a doctor may, for ethical reasons, withhold advice which is legally permissible. The Ethical Committee of the British Medical Association, for example, has not altered its code of practice to allow full implementation of the 1967 Abortion Act. It is interesting then that in commenting on the Act the Catholic Bishops of England and Wales stated, 'It is not part of a doctor's duty to impose his ethical views on his patients. He should however explain to a patient seeking an abortion why he is unable to co-operate.' It is agreed by Roman Catholic lawyers that a doctor who has a conscientious objection to therapeutic abortion should refer the patient to another doctor.

If two or more doctors have the care of the same patient it is in the patient's interest that they should communicate as freely as possible. Some contraceptive procedures are so simple that, if a woman seeks advice from a specialist in this field, the doctor need not always feel obliged to inform any others who may have care of the patient. However, the practice has grown up, in Britain at any rate, of communicating with the woman's doctor before giving the Pill. The patient's doctor should be informed when an IUD is inserted and in the case of sterilization or abortion all who have medical care of the family will be deeply involved and constructive advice from other doctors is of the utmost value.

When oral contraceptives are given the prescribing doctor, if he is not the patient's own practitioner, should communicate with the latter to discover if there is any medical contra-indication and in order to inform him that a prescription has been issued. In some instances, especially in the case of the unmarried or the divorced, the patient may refuse permission for the prescribing doctor to communicate with her own practitioner. When this situation arises the doctor should try to persuade the patient otherwise, but his first duty is to the patient seeking advice and the possibility of withholding a prescription should not be used as a threat; the case should be judged only on medical grounds. If a doctor has moral objections to the use of contraceptives, either generally or in particular circumstances, he may explain his point of view to a patient but he cannot refuse to allow another doctor to prescribe the Pill, fit an IUD or advise on any other method of contraception.

CONSENT

1 Contraceptives

In English law coitus interruptus, the use of a sheath and intercourse following vasectomy have been held to constitute consummation of a marriage.[10] Some caution may be required in prescribing oral contraceptives if the husband is known to disapprove but the doctor's liability in such cases is probably very small.[11]

If contraceptive advice is given to a girl under the age of consent (16 years in England) it could be construed as aiding and abetting a criminal act, even if the consent of the patient and her parents is obtained. The practitioner would be wise to secure legal advice in such cases. Any ruling would, of course, not apply to a doctor using orally active progestagen and oestrogen compounds in the treatment of dysmenorrhea or other menstrual symptoms.

The written consent of both partners should be obtained before inserting an IUD and there should be some record that the patient is aware of the risks of the method. If the husband's consent is not available the doctor should proceed with some caution. An intrauterine device may still be used if there is a medical contra-indication to further pregnancies, but the doctor would be advised to take legal advice as a husband has a right to the opportunity of having children.

2 Sterilization

Normally the written consent of the man and woman is essential before surgical sterilization for either sex. Legal advice must be taken before operating if the patient is thought to be mentally defective and cannot fully understand the nature of the operation or if the consent of the sexual partner is not available.

In questionable cases, when legal advice has been obtained, the opinion of a second practitioner could also be of value, and in all cases it is important to keep clear, detailed records.

3 Abortion

The written consent of the patient must be obtained, but under the English Abortion Act 1967 the consent of the husband is not obligatory, though it is prudent to have the husband's consent whenever possible. The doctor should ensure that when the patient gives her consent she is not being subjected to undue pressure. If the girl is under 21 the parents should be consulted whenever possible, but only with the patient's consent. Girls under 16 are an exception and the parents must be consulted; nevertheless it remains legally proper to terminate the pregnancy even if the parents of the girl withhold consent whether she is under 21 or under 16 years of age.

The doctor's responsibility is two-way and he could be considered liable for negligence if a woman died as a result of his failure to operate.

When dealing with the after-effects of an illegal abortion the doctor is not legally bound to disclose information discovered during the course of his medical duties.

THE EFFECTIVENESS OF LEGISLATION

It was the unanimous view of the 1957 Wolfenden Committee that 'it is not the function of the law to intervene in the private lives of citizens or to seek to enforce any particular pattern of behaviour'. The attempt to do so in the field of reproductive behaviour is especially futile; in the long run the law comes to be held in contempt and in the meantime the consequences of evasion can be socially disastrous. This is certainly the case in relation to the statutory regulation of contraception, sterilization and abortion in societies which, at the same time, give lip-service to the validity of individual judgement.

No country can effectively legislate against contraception if parents wish to limit their families; the most widely used form of contraception requires the existence of neither manufacturer, advertiser nor point of sale—and it costs nothing. On the other hand, it is not amongst the most reliable forms of birth control, and the effect of outlawing alternatives is simply to condemn parents to a technique which is second best. And because termination is an obvious longstop to contraceptive failure the demand for abortion, which in these circumstances is only likely to be available illegally, will be high.

This is exactly the set of circumstances which has prevailed in France but, at different levels, it is paralleled wherever free and unimpeded access to contraception (including sterilization) is denied. The state laws of Connecticut and Massachusetts, for example, would be of little importance (since contraceptives are commercially available and doctors will prescribe privately) if they did not prevent the establishment of birth control clinics. The consequence is that the better methods of contraception are denied to precisely those parents who need them most.

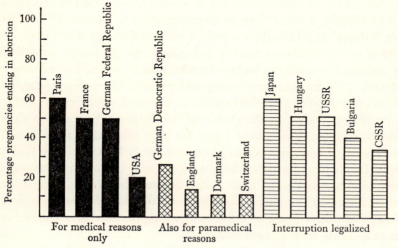

Fig. 37. Abortion rates (legal and illegal) and abortion law regulations in various countries, 1966.

Thus, although the extent of contraceptive practice in any society cannot be inferred from the presence or absence of restricting legislation, the quality, effectiveness and consequent safety of available techniques will be directly related to the degree of freedom which the law allows. Similarly the scale of liberality of the law on abortion is no indication of the prevalence of abortion in a community. Figure 37 demonstrates that there are countries in which abortion is unequivocally illegal which show rates of termination quite as high as those prevailing in some of the countries where interruption is legalized and those countries which have attempted a partial liberalization of the law show, on balance, lower rates than countries where the law remains unchanged. The sole predictable effect of legislation is to determine the relative ratio of 'illegal' and 'legal' terminations amongst an otherwise predetermined total. In practice, as in theory, this may be a merely semantic distinction as in Britain and America.

In these countries the abortion situation represents the classic illustration of patterned evasion—statutory insistence on standards of behaviour which are systematically contravened in practice. Because the law prohibits clinical termination women seeking abortion are driven to obtain it by illegal means; the fact that abortion then comes to be regarded as 'criminal' in turn makes reform of the law more difficult. Yet, despite the fact that there are at least 40,000 illegal abortions a year in Britain, a mere fifty prosecutions result. There can be few other 'crimes' in which the committal rate is as low as 1 in 1,000.

But if governments are unable to legislate against family limitation they are equally unable to impose standards of reproductive behaviour by decree. This, too, has been attempted by regimes pursuing pronatalist policies but it has not met with noticeable success. Equally, governments can be wrong-headed in the choice of family planning methods they choose to support. The case of Japan has been referred to already, and there are other countries which have learnt only by experience that a rational family planning policy involves free access to all forms of contraception and to abortion as a last resort. Beyond this it is an exercise in public education to convince individuals of the value of family planning and to create the climate of opinion in which personal convenience is seen to coincide with general welfare.

VOLUNTARY ORGANIZATIONS

When the law becomes manifestly out of step with social needs the opportunity is created, in democratic societies, for the formation of pressure groups. Voluntary organizations of this kind have a basic commitment to changing the law but, as one means to this end, they may also undertake to do what the state refuses to condone or to accept as public responsibility. This was the function of the birth control movements in England and America which, in addition to their propagandist and educational activities, have provided an administrative framework later to become a model for public authority subvention. Birth control provision in England was never illegal and the clinics were able to operate unhindered by the law. In the US, on the other hand, the early clinics were also challenging the law; Mrs Sanger's clinics were closed down by the police in 1916 and again in 1929[12] but since that date there has been no further interference with the activities of the Planned Parenthood Leagues except in Massachusetts and Connecticut.

Voluntary bodies attempting to popularize sterilization (or, more accurately, to remove public misconception and resolve legal ambiguity) have obviously made less progress than the birth control movements. Sterilization has been a more emotive topic than contraception and until recently the major organizations concerned, the Human Betterment Association of America and the Eugenics Society and Simon Population Trust in England, have attempted to operate by stealth rather than by publicity. In the more favourable circumstances which they have thus created both the Human Betterment Association and the Simon Population Trust now feel able to act as agencies for individuals requesting surgical sterilization. The former organization maintains a roster of 1,100 co-operating physicians in the US to one of whom enquirers are directed by the social worker in charge. In 1966 the Simon Population Trust established a project whose primary aim is to promote male sterilization by assisting volunteers to obtain the necessary surgical treatment.[13] An important feature of the scheme is the close liaison which is maintained with the family doctor with whom the final decision in a particular case always rests; for this reason the Trust is not always informed of the outcome of cases which it has initiated, but in the first year of operation nearly 1,000 vaso-ligations were carried out.

The Abortion Law Reform Association in England was largely instrumental in obtaining the changes embodied in the 1967 Act.[14] Though these represented only a part of what the Association had demanded, with the passing of the Act an immediate need was created for ensuring that its provisions were fully utilized. For this purpose, voluntary workers in London and in Birmingham have established Pregnancy Advisory Services to assist women who are in a state of distress as a result of becoming pregnant. The aims of the services, whose telephone numbers can be obtained through the municipal information bureaux in the cities concerned, are 'to provide advice, treatment and assistance for women who are suffering from any physical or mental illness or distress as a result of or during pregnancy, including such medical, psychiatric or other treatment as may be required in connection with the lawful termination of pregnancy and otherwise in the alleviation or relief of such illness or distress with power to establish and operate (whether alone or in co-operation with any other body or individual) clinics or medical centres for the benefit of such persons'.

In the international field much of the credit for the spread of family planning during the last twenty years belongs to the voluntary International Planned Parenthood Federation. This organization was formed at the international conference convened by Margaret Sanger in 1948 (see p. 16); originally named the International Committee on Planned Parenthood it adopted its present title in 1952. The Federation is an association of national family planning associations and a number of governmental organizations have affiliate membership. By conducting research, publishing a range of scientific literature and organizing international conferences the IPPF has obtained recognition as the authority on all aspects of family limitation. The Federation has consultative status with the United Nations Organization, the World Health Organization and the Food and Agriculture Organization. The American Population Council (see p. 36) also relies on both voluntary and governmental funds to finance its research, publications and fertility control programmes in developing countries.

15 MEDICAL ASPECTS

The doctor giving family planning advice has a unique and valuable opportunity to practise in a number of spheres. He will meet a wide range of gynaecological conditions, he can take an important part in preventive medicine, he can be a counsellor in marital and sexual problems and, quite properly, he can get drawn into the wider practice of social medicine. Conversely, where the British ideal of general practice exists the family doctor is almost always the best placed to give contraceptive advice.

GYNAECOLOGY

1 Vaginal and cervical conditions

Vaginitis and cervicitis are so common that many women accept them as part of the marital state and a vaginal discharge, like wearing a wedding ring, is assumed to be universal. A discharge which may take one woman to a hospital outpatients may go unheeded in her neighbour. The family planning doctor must use the opportunities he is given to improve the health and comfort of his patients without at the same time seeking perfection by treating minor conditions which have not given symptoms and, anyhow, will relapse after therapy.

The healthy vagina has a thin serous secretion which is just sufficient to lubricate it. The vagina is at pH 4 to 5 due to fermentation of the glycogen in the desquamated epithelial cells by Döderlein's bacillus. When *Trichomonas vaginalis* is present lactobacilli are rarely found and the pH is raised. There is a creamy, yellow, slightly frothy vaginal discharge, the vaginal walls may be red and inflamed and there may be pruritis, dyspareunia and frequency of micturition. The diagnosis can be confirmed by mixing a drop of the discharge with saline and examining the unstained preparation under a microscope. *Trichomonas* is pear-shaped, slightly larger than a leucocyte, it has four flagellae, an axostyle, an undulatory membrane and is best observed when motile.

Trichomonas infestation is a venereal disease in that it is most usually transmitted by sexual intercourse and the organism often infects the sexual partner. Although there is sometimes a urethritis, the male infection is commonly asymptomatic.

The amount of glycogen in the epithelial cells, and therefore the vaginal pH, depends on the level of circulating oestrogens and *Trichomonas* infection may be aggravated by oral contraceptives and it may be worth changing to a preparation with a higher oestrogen content (page 97).

Both partners should be given metronidazole (Flagyl) 200 mg three times a day for seven days. The course can be repeated if necessary. Metronidazole has practically no side effects and only very rarely have toxic rashes (and possibly leucopenia) been reported. The use of a condom cuts down the risk of infection from a male carrier of *Trichomonas*.

Infection with the fungus *Candida albicans*—vaginal thrush—is slightly less widespread than *Trichomonas* but still common. The vaginal discharge is white and cheesy and adherent white patches may be seen on speculum examination. Pruritis and dyspareunia are more intense than in most *Trichomonas* infections. The organism can be quite difficult to demonstrate and smears must be Gram stained. *Candida* infection may be a presenting symptom of diabetes mellitus and the urine should be tested for glycosuria.

Thrush can be persistent and the patient must understand that any treatment should be carried out for the prescribed time and not discontinued as soon as symptoms have subsided. Nystatin or candicidin pessaries or ointment (twice daily for 14 days) should be used. Painting the vagina with 1 per cent gentian violet solution, while exceedingly messy and rarely used, can be useful in overcoming an obstinate infection.

Chronic cervicitis is common and troublesome. Usually there is an offensive discharge but pruritis is uncommon. The cervix appears inflamed when examined with a speculum, there may be some Nabothian follicles and sometimes frank ulceration. Cauterization may be necessary. If an IUD is to be fitted cervicitis should be treated before insertion whenever possible.

Cervical polypi are sometimes found when the cervix is visualized with a speculum. Often they will have been asymptomatic but sometimes there will have been a history of post-coital bleeding. A polyp can be twisted off as an office procedure, although cervical dilatation and cautery may be appropriate in some cases. The specimen should always be examined histologically.

The stratified squamous epithelium of the vagina changes abruptly to columnar epithelium at a point just proximal to the external cervical os. The junction is a zone of some instability and columnar epithelium, by a process of migration or metaplasia, may be found outside the os constituting an erosion. Sometimes an erosion is associated with cervicitis but on many occasions it is asymptomatic and requires no treatment. Erosions commonly regress spontaneously and, unless complicated by infection, do not constitute a contra-indication to any form of contraception.

2   Venereal disease

Acute gonorrhoea presents as a prurulent urethritis and cervicitis, but this is rare and the disease is more commonly diagnosed from the history or by microscopy. A primary syphilitic chancre is even rarer and again the diagnosis is usually made in other ways.

Any proved or suspected case of venereal disease demands treatment in a specialist centre both because partial and unsatisfactory treatment is dangerous and because special skills are needed in following up contacts.

3   Other conditions

Gynaecological complaints, from congenital abnormalities to malignancy, may be discovered during history taking or when performing a pelvic examination. Almost always the patient will have to be referred for specialist advice. While a small proportion of patients who seek advice on family planning will find themselves passed on to a gynaecologist, it is to be hoped that a large number of women who have gynaecological or obstetric treatment will be given, or referred for, contraceptive care. A question on contraception is often the most important part of a routine post-natal examination.

PREVENTIVE MEDICINE

It is a prerequisite of good medical care that the doctor understands his various roles clearly and is able to distinguish between them. He must have a positive idea when and why he wants to see his patient again.

Women on oral contraceptives are often seen unnecessarily frequently and for confused reasons. Sometimes there are pharmaceutical regulations which prevent prescription for longer than a year, but there are no medical reasons why a healthy woman should be seen at all frequently once she is settled on a suitable preparation. Thrombosis cannot be diagnosed in advance, weight gain will bring the woman back herself if she is worried and so will changes in the pattern of menstruation. Episodes of cerebral insufficiency have been reported in one individual woman which might have been an effect of Pill-induced thrombosis, but it is not a condition that can be subject to routine screening. It is a waste of time to see a woman three-monthly, as is often done, and can lead to unnecessary worry for the patient. The patient may need to be seen six-monthly if she cannot afford to buy many cycles at a time or loses her prescription, but once yearly is sufficiently adequate on purely medical grounds. Greater flexibility in timing follow-up visits is necessary when an IUD is fitted and a careful history and pelvic examination may detect a previously unrecognized pelvic infection. Also, some women will persist with an IUD when it is not in their medical interest to do so; for example, they may have become severely anaemic.

IUD check visits or the giving of Pill prescriptions can be used as a convenient reason to recall women for routine measures of preventive medicine such as cervical cytology and breast examination. The doctor —and usually the patient—should understand what is being done and that the examination is not directly related to her method of contraception. It should also be remembered that routine visits concerning a diaphragm, or any other method of contraception, may be used in the same way (see p. 119).

One-third of all deaths among women aged 15 to 44 are due to neoplasia and once a doctor has advised a satisfactory method of contraception any possible side effects due to the woman's contraceptive method may, with justice, take second place to commonsense steps in preventive medicine. The family planning doctor may be the only physician that the woman sees with any regularity and a cervical smear and question on lumps in the breast can be life-saving. Women of high parity and low social class are most at risk for cervical cancer—and least likely to volunteer for the examination (see p. 119).

The incidence of cervical carcinoma in situ and microinvasive carcinoma is maximal 10 to 19 years after first coitus. In a normal urban population the incidence of preclinical cancer detected by cervical smears rises from under 0·05 per cent in the 20 to 25 age-group to over 1 per cent in the 40 to 45 age-group. The British Ministry of Health (1965) recommended screening women aged 35 to 60 at five-yearly intervals, but three-yearly screening beginning at the age of 25 is an ideal some cytohistopathologists would like to achieve.

When taking a Papanicolaou smear an unlubricated speculum should be passed before any digital examination is made. Material should be collected from the posterior fornix and from the cervix using the two ends (Y-shaped end for the cervix) of a disposable wooden spatula, spread evenly on a labelled glassed slide and fixed immediately. It is important not to allow the cells to dry in the air. The slides should be fixed for 15 min and may then be drained and stored dry. The cytological laboratory usually provides a form to be filled in when the specimens are taken.

In British Columbia, where cytological services have been operating since 1949, one-third of fertile women are screened for cervical cancer and incidence of clinically invasive cancer has fallen from 28·4 to 19·7 per thousand.[1]

When possible the breasts should be examined and the woman taught to palpate her own breasts, especially if the patient is over 35. In Britain the average size of the lump which women discover is over 3 cm in diameter and by this time 50 per cent of malignancies have metastases.

After malignancies the next most common causes of death in fertile women are accidents, poisoning and violence. A proportion of these deaths are, one way or another, related to the tyranny of excess fertility and the family planning doctor is fortunate in being able to contribute to the health of society on a wide front.

PROBLEMS OF SEXUAL BEHAVIOUR

When a doctor gives contraceptive advice he enters a very private sphere of human experience. He must understand the patient in order to adopt an attitude which ensures that the relevant technical information gets across and he should have a lively awareness of the numerous emotional problems of courtship, marriage and sexual behaviour which may find expression in a couple's attitude to contraception. The time when birth control is received may be used as the moment when help is sought for a wide range of social and psychological problems. However, few marriages are perfect and the range of human sexual behaviour so boundless that those who look for problems must expect to discover many. There is nothing to be gained and much to be lost if premarital or marital difficulties are uncovered without giving any constructive help. Any articulate questioner can very easily unearth examples of sexual maladjustment but relatively few are able to offer really wise counsel, and some problems must be recognized as socially or psychologically incurable.

The doctor must understand his own attitudes and responsibilities before he can help the patient. Intimate questions on sexual behaviour should only be asked if the doctor has a specific purpose in mind. The doctor must avoid idle curiosity, or worse, the vicarious satisfaction of his or her own sexual interest. A carefully thought out investigation of sexual behaviour can produce invaluable information but routine questions to every woman seeking contraceptive advice, such as frequency of coitus, are purposeless. On the whole, intimate questions are more acceptable when they are asked by a doctor than by lay assistants or nurses—although there can be important exceptions to this generalization.

When advice is given it can be at two levels. Most doctors have the experience to offer commonsense advice for commonplace problems. It is important to remember that the barriers to communication between social groups are greatest in the realm of sexual behaviour and advice must be translated into appropriate language: on the one hand sexual intercourse may need to be described in terms of Anglo–Saxon philology and common medical terms such as 'the menopause' are meaningless to some patients; on the other, condescending chats about 'the front passage' can be equally out of place for a sophisticated woman.

When possible, complex problems should be referred for specialist advice: the gynaecological couch must not be confused with the psychiatric couch. The more disturbed the patient or the more difficult her social circumstances the greater will be the need for adequate contraceptive advice, and it may be necessary to avoid probing questions in order to retain her co-operation. Sometimes little history, or even the name or age of the sexual partner, may be obtained without risk of loss of confidence and it may be necessary to sacrifice the physical examination so that the patient may feel at ease. A woman who has confidence in her adviser can be seen more often than usual and a rapport developed which allows long-term help to be given.

ADVICE FOR THE UNMARRIED

Contraceptive advice to the unmarried is still a controversial subject, and although the heat of debate of former years has now died down concerning contraception for the married, the embers can still be reignited when advice is given to the young unmarried. It is often forgotten that the condom has been available to the married and unmarried for many years, and to prescribe the Pill for, say, an unmarried student is not to do anything new except to make a more effective method available.

The age of marriage is declining in all developed nations and whereas 48,000 brides were under the age of 21 in England and Wales in 1921 the number was 152,000 in 1965. Correspondingly, young people are beginning sexual exploration at a younger age, and in a sample of nearly 2,000 young people Schofield[2] found that 30 per cent of boys and 16 per cent of girls aged 17 to 19 had had sexual intercourse. Often there is some interval between episodes of sexual experiment and in a significant number of cases the second intercourse takes place with a different partner. There are no outstanding features in the home background or social environment which distinguish those who have premarital sexual experience: they are anybody's and everybody's son or daughter.

In Schofield's study less than half the boys and only one-fifth of the girls always used contraceptives and a quarter of the boys and nearly two-thirds of the girls never used contraceptives. The condom, of course, is used most widely.

In Britain in 1964 two out of three girls marrying under the age of 20 were pregnant and 22 per cent of all births under 20 were illegitimate. Early marriages are less stable and in the United States the divorce rate is treble the average for girls marrying under 20 years of age.[3] Women who marry young have more children than average both because their fertility is higher and because they are exposed to the risk of pregnancy for more years.

When contraceptive advice is made available to the unmarried the majority of couples who accept it have been having sexual relations for three months to one year and less than 5 per cent of the girls seeking advice are virgins. Most have a stable relationship and many marry quite soon.

It is in the clear interest of both society and the individual to make contraceptive advice available to the unmarried as well as the married. It does not lead to promiscuity, but it may prevent some unwanted pregnancies and enable some more mature and responsible marriages to take place.

It is important to use the most effective and acceptable method, and oral contraceptives are nearly always the first choice. Paradoxically, the closeness of the general practitioner's bonds with the family unit may conflict with the young person's desire for anonymity, and the patient may forgo advice she desperately needs rather than discuss the problem with the doctor 'who knows my parents', or who has been a very real friend since childhood. The young person often wishes to turn to another doctor or a specialist clinic.

Possibly greater wisdom and understanding are needed when advising the unmarried than the married and certainly they will have their share of psychological illness, but it is misleading to imagine, as some have done, that every unmarried person who seeks contraceptive advice may be emotionally disturbed.

EARLY DIAGNOSIS OF PREGNANCY

Pregnancy is the commonest cause of sudden cessation of menstruation in a healthy woman of the fertile years and when this symptom presents in the context of giving family planning advice the diagnosis is even more likely. The commonest alternative diagnosis of a delayed period is an alteration in the woman's pattern of menstruation. Such an alteration is often said to follow a change of environment or some psychological stress, but it must be remembered that variation in cycle length in an individual is common. On very rare occasions amenorrhea may be associated with thyroid dysfunction or a complication of a specific infection.

Uterine enlargement can be felt on bimanual pelvic examination between six and eight weeks of pregnancy. The fundus generally feels round and cystic, the cervix soft and 'velvety' to touch. The uterus can be palpated abdominally at about twelve weeks in primigravidae and sometimes a little earlier in a multiparous patient. It is midway between the symphisis pubis and umbilicus by the sixteenth week of pregnancy.

In the first six to eight weeks of pregnancy diagnosis is uncertain and pregnancy tests are of great value. Some women have a conviction that they are pregnant, which should not be dismissed lightly. Frequency of micturation is common between six and ten weeks, nausea may begin about the time of the first missed period and breast discomfort, of the type experienced premenstrually, may also appear at about four weeks and persist for some time. Breast changes such as pigmentation and increased prominence of Montgomery's tubercles and a characteristic dusky discolouration of the vaginal mucosa and cervix often appear in the second month.

A great many biochemical and cytological changes occur during pregnancy. The cervical mucus undergoes cyclical alterations in weight, sodium and protein content and the viscosity vary dramatically. Cervical mucus can be drawn into long stringy threads at the time of ovulation, but if a blob of mucus is placed between a slide and cover-slip in early pregnancy it is difficult to separate the two and the mucus adheres to one surface.[4] When cervical mucus collected at the time of ovulation dries on a slide it crystallizes into patterns resembling fern leaves, but under the influence of progesterone, as in early pregnancy, it dries without any ferning or arborization.

The most certain and widely used tests of early pregnancy involve detecting chorionic gonadotrophin. Human chorionic gonadotrophin (HCG) is first detectable in the serum and urine between the twenty-first and twenty-fifth day of pregnancy and it reaches to maximum in the second and third months. It is mainly luteinizing in type—a fact used in the Hogben test when human urinary gonadotrophins injected into female *Xenopus laevis* causes ovulation. Immunological assays are simpler and cheaper than biological tests and are more widely used. The urine from the woman requesting the pregnancy test is mixed with antisera produced by injecting HCG into a rabbit. If the woman is pregnant the urinary HCG reacts with the antisera. However, there is insufficient HCG in pregnant urine to produce a visible precipitate and a second step is necessary to visualize that a reaction has occurred. Either sheep red cells sensitized to HCG (Pregnosticon test) or latex particles coated with HCG (Gravindex test) are added to the mixed urine and rabbit antisera. If there was no HCG in the urine to react with the antisera then the sheep cells or latex particles will be agglutinated, but if the patient was pregnant they will remain dispersed. The Gravindex test takes two minutes and can be performed on a slide.

Immunological tests are positive in 95 per cent of cases[5] and false positives do not normally occur, although albuminurea and a history of ingestion of phenothiazines should be eliminated. Pregnancy tests may be positive within a week of the first missed period, although a negative result is no proof pregnancy has not occurred and the test should be repeated a week later.

If menstruation is delayed in the absence of pregnancy then uterine bleeding can usually be induced by giving a progesterone/oestrogen combination for a few days and then withdrawing it. Five milligrams norethisterone and 0·01 mg ethinylestradiol (Primodos) on two successive days or 10 mg dimesthisterone and 0·05 ethylestradiol (Secrodyl) twice daily for two days are suitable preparations.

THE SUBFERTILE COUPLE

Although the precise proportion of the married population who will, in the future, seek the help of doctors in limiting their families may be speculative, it is certain that most of that minority of couples who find themselves involuntarily childless will regard this as a matter for medical consultation. Virtually all couples enter marriage with an expectation of becoming parents and sterility is perhaps a more distressing phenomenon to the individuals concerned than excess fertility. In relation to the prevailing stereotype of ideal family size non-fulfilment, as well as over-achievement, is regarded as deviant behaviour and social norms are, in this context, reinforced by psychological feelings of inadequacy or even of guilt which may, in their turn, adversely affect the marriage relationship. On the other hand the marriage may, for other reasons, be unsuccessful and the doctor should be sceptical about the couple who seek to hasten pregnancy in the naïve belief that the arrival of a child will in itself improve the relationship.

The literature on subfertility is vast, and, as with many other disciplines, there appears to be an inverse relationship between the large volume of published work and the very modest degree of practical achievement. The aetiology of subfertility in men and women is obscure; only in a relatively small proportion of cases is an accurate diagnosis possible and even for these there is no definitive form of treatment. In a volume which is primarily concerned with contraception only the most cursory review of the major diagnostic and remedial procedures is necessary—sufficient to enable the non-specialist to cope with the enquiries of patients and to be familiar with the nature and range of specialist help on which he may call. For a more extensive treatment the reader is referred to one of the standard texts.[6,7]

1 Definition

The inability to conceive is variously referred to as sterility, subfertility, infecundity, barrenness and infertility. By convention the sterm *sterility* is used of those couples in whom the inability to conceive is apparently irremediable and *subfertility* or infertility (which has a different connotation in demography and sociology) of those for whom conception is theoretically possible. It is the latter which constitutes the ongoing concern of the family planning doctor and subfertility may be either *primary*, implying that conception has never occurred, or *secondary*, denoting that there have been earlier pregnancies but further conception cannot be achieved. The American Society for the Study of Sterility has attempted to provide a generic definition by suggesting that a marriage may be regarded as infertile, and thus appropriate for investigation, 'when pregnancy has not occurred after a year of coitus without contraception'.

2 Extent

The precise extent of biological infecundity in any population is difficult to assess. Demographic data makes no distinction between voluntary and involuntary childlessness and couples ignorant of their infecundity may be revealed as contraceptive-users in sociological enquiries. The Indianapolis Study estimated that 9·8 per cent of American couples interviewed were involuntarily childless and the Royal Commission on Population suggested that 7 per cent of English marriages were biologically infertile. Other investigators, in both countries, have arrived at broadly comparable estimates.

3 Aetiology and Diagnosis

Although infertility is usually regarded as a gynaecological problem and it is usually the woman who first seeks clinical help, in only 50 per cent of cases does the fault lie with the woman; in 30 per cent of couples the husband is responsible and in the remaining 20 per cent the problem is mutual and each partner might prove fecund within another union.

Subfertility in men may result either from seminal defects or from the inability to deposit semen in such a position that spermatozoa, in sufficient quantity to produce conception, are able to enter the cervix. In women the aetiology is more complex and includes anatomical defects of the vagina and cervix or excessive cervical secretions preventing the entry of spermatozoa; endometrial malfunctioning resulting in the inability of the uterus to allow nidation, repeated spontaneous abortions, failure of ovulation (which may be due to pituitary or ovarian defects) and occlusion of the Fallopian tubes. The diagnostic routine is designed to facilitate the progressive elimination of each of these possible sources of infecundity.

(a) CASE HISTORY

A careful and painstaking history of both partners should be separately obtained. This should include previous operations and illnesses (including venereal disease which is unlikely to be divulged in a joint interview), reproductive experience in earlier unions and, in the case of the woman, details of her menstrual history. The marital record, including the frequency and timing of coitus, may provide clues which make further investigation unnecessary. It is frequently discovered that couples who have come to suspect their subfecundity have, in an attempt to conceive, confined coitus to the menstrual phase of the cycle as a result of erroneous information derived from friends or from books.

(b) PHYSICAL EXAMINATION

In the woman, scarring may confirm or contradict details of previous operations obtained during interview; hirsutism may be suggestive of endocrinological disorders and a pelvic examination should reveal any anatomical obstacle to impregnation. Hypospadias and urethral stricture are the most commonly occurring physical defects in the male.

(c) PHYSIOLOGICAL TESTS

These are designed to evaluate, in the male and in the female respectively, the ability to produce viable sperm and the ability to produce a fertilizable ovum and to retain it after impregnation. Semen testing is a routine microscopic procedure which takes account of sperm density, morphology and motility and testicular biopsy may prove useful. Daily recording of basal body temperature (see chapter 8) is the most convenient means of ascertaining if and when ovulation takes place; this test will be substantiated by information regarding mid-cycle bleeding or *mittelschmerz* in some patients. Endometrial biopsy provides information on the endometrial response to ovulation and the ovarian hormones.

(d) ANATOMICAL TESTS

These usually include the post-coital test, designed to ascertain the degree of sperm invasion of the cervix by microscopic examination of cervical mucous carried out three to eight hours after intercourse together with an assessment of tubal patency by insufflation of the tubes with carbon dioxide during which a kymograph tracing records both patency and peristalsis. Salpingohysterography, involving the instillation into the cervix of radio-opaque fluid, instead of carbon dioxide, and subsequent X-ray photography is occasionally preferred to the latter since it may also reveal pathological defects in the endometrial cavity.

(e) PSYCHOLOGICAL FACTORS

An important index of the immaturity of a discipline is the extent to which it relies on psychological explanations for non-psychological events. The frequency with which psychological, psychiatric and 'psychogenic' factors are invoked as an explanation of subfertility is no more than an indication of the insecurity of its practitioners. In a critical[8] analysis of seventy-five selected papers on psychological factors affecting fertility Noyes and Chapnick have shown that no fewer than fifty different factors were postulated! The various authors assumed, or even stated, that psychological factors altered fertility *per se*, though no conclusive evidence was ever offered, and the reviewers comment on the very scant use of evidence, its poor presentation and on the unsystematic quoting of the literature. Even in a standard, and otherwise highly respectable, work Buxton and Southam state, 'there *must* be psychogenic factors as an actual cause of infertility' but the only diagnostic procedure recommended is 'intuition'. This appears to be a particularly unfruitful approach to what is generally an obscure physiological problem.

4   Therapy

The precise mode of treatment will depend upon the findings in each individual case and some defects are more amenable to therapy than others. The available techniques include hormonal therapy or the use of clomiphene designed to bring about the maturation and release of ovarian follicles, the systematic confinement of coitus to the ovulatory phase, hydrotubation and tuboplasty, with artificial insemination as a last resort. Hormone therapy has proved singularly ineffective in azoospermic and oligospermic males. Caution should be exercised in attempting subfertility treatment of the habitual aborting woman in cases where this is not clearly the result of cervical incompetence. At least 20 per cent of spontaneous abortions have gross chromosomal aberrations.

5 Evaluation

It is virtually impossible to evaluate the individual techniques of sub-fertility treatment by the usual canons of scientific validity because

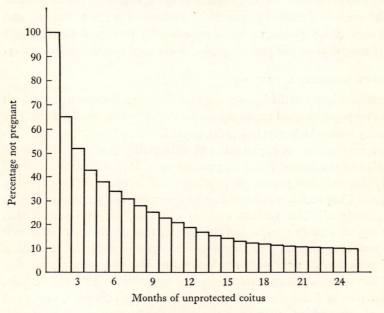

Fig. 38. Percentage of women remaining non-pregnant after varying periods of marriage.

normal experimental procedures (including double-blind testing) are not applicable. The work of subfertility clinics is usually justified in terms of the overall success rate achieved, and one investigator has revealingly suggested that 'thorough and methodical investigation is therapy in itself'.[9] There may, however, be a simpler explanation for the apparent success of subfertility investigation. The average time required for conception is illustrated graphically in figure 38 which is based on accumulated data from clinical and demographic studies; if the ASSS definition is adopted as a working hypothesis (and most couples do seek clinical help during the first year) then the rate of spontaneous cure will be about 50 per cent.

16 A CONSPECTUS

THE STATUS OF CONTRACEPTIVE PRACTICE

Contraception is a relatively recent but increasingly important medical specialism. As if to compensate for the long delay in admitting it to the curriculum it is now afforded undisputed recognition, and national or international conferences can attract platform support from amongst the most eminent members of the medical profession. Like most of the specialist disciplines which have reached maturity during recent years conception control is an eclectic enterprise, drawing on the literature and techniques of the physiology of reproduction, obstetric surgery and endocrinology as well as on the findings and theories of sociology and demography. Its location, amongst that range of medical and para-medical activities which form the major growth point in contemporary preventive medicine and through which general practice will become more closely integrated with specialist treatment and research, is both unique and ubiquitous. Childbirth may be the one surgical procedure which virtually every woman can expect to undergo (though abortion has been shown to be a strong challenger in many countries), but the spacing and limitation of births is also a universal need.

Contraception's earlier dubiety has also been replaced by a glamour of sorts. The Pill is regarded by the public as one of the major scientific discoveries of the present century, the IUD has an apparently continuing fascination for the layman and any future development is assured of an appreciative reception. Concern over the world population explosion has added a further dimension to public interest in birth control. Contraception, in western societies, is concerned with the fun end of the reproductive process and thus constitutes an obvious target for the moralizing critics of affluence and permissiveness, but on the world scale it is seen to be a humanitarian pursuit of unprecedented importance. Nor can it be too often stressed that effective fertility control programmes and techniques in underdeveloped countries will depend very largely on the experience of advanced societies.

To the doctor working in an English or American city the problem of world population growth may seem remote and he may wish to evaluate his activities in the field of conception control by reference to its more immediate contribution to individual well-being and community welfare. In preventive medicine these latter are indistinguishable ends and their interrelationships, extending as they may over two or more generations, preclude accurate statistical assessment. Nevertheless, a number of important points have emerged in previous chapters which merit review.

PREVENTIVE MEDICINE AND PUBLIC HEALTH

The correlation between excessive childbearing, poverty and family ill-health is familiar to every doctor with a working-class practice and is reflected in a wide range of official statistics and epidemiological studies.

1 Maternal Morbidity and Mortality

The maternal mortality rate is defined as the number of women dying from delivery or complications of pregnancy, childbirth or puerperium (but excluding deaths from abortion) during one year per 1,000 live births and stillbirths in the same period. The maternal morbidity rate is the number of women suffering from diseases attributable to the same causes per 1,000 women of the same age-group. Both are important indices of the general health of the community. The incidence of a large number of diseases including anaemia, postpartum haemorrhage and placenta praevia have been shown to increase with parity and almost every other disease can only be aggravated by uncontrolled fertility. The risk of death through the complications of childbirth and the puerperium has been enormously reduced in western societies during the last sixty years. Yet there are wide differences in the rates for specific groups and these are found to be more closely related to age than to other social variables. Age and parity are highly correlated and, on the basis of special tabulations made available by the Registrar General, Benjamin[1] has shown that within every age-group there is a high risk at first maternity, a low risk at second and third and beyond this the risk increases with increasing parity until it reaches and exceeds the level prevailing for first maternities.

2   Abortion

Although deaths due to abortion are excluded from maternal mortality statistics the role of abortion, especially of criminal abortion, as a cause of maternal death has already been noted. In the Confidential Enquiry into Maternal Deaths in England and Wales in 1961–3,[2] abortion was revealed as the commonest single cause of death, the majority of cases following illegal interruption of pregnancy; in New York, during 1958–60 the proportion of maternal deaths associated with abortion, again predominantly illegal, was 43·6 per cent.[3] There is external evidence that a high proportion of these were multiparous women. In some Latin American countries abortion is the commonest cause of death among women of fertile years and not merely a component of maternal mortality.

It has been argued in this volume that acceptance of the principle of contraception must also entail an acceptance of abortion as a final defence against unwanted pregnancy. Yet, because of the inadequacy of existing contraceptive facilities, abortion is too frequently a method of first resort. Abortion has been described as the greatest epidemic of all time; certainly it absorbs a disproportionate share of scarce medical resources and, in terms of its contribution to maternal mortality and morbidity, is amongst the least desirable forms of birth control. Termination should be a once-for-all experience for any particular women if those entrusted with her medical care are acting rationally and conscientiously.

3   Low Birth Weight Prematurity

Prematurity is internationally defined in terms of a birth weight of less than 2,500 g (5½ lb) irrespective of the period of gestation which in many societies cannot be estimated and even in societies with fully developed maternity services can be accurately assessed in only 80 to 90 per cent of births. The rate of prematurity is usually expressed as a percentage of all live births and the prevailing rate in Britain is 7 per cent.

There is a large literature relating low birth weight to subsequent defects in physical[4] and intellectual[5] development; equally well established is the relationship between prematurity and other variables amongst which parity, marital status and social class are the most influential. In a large-scale study in Edinburgh during 1953–4[6] class differentials in the incidence of prematurity were mediated by parity. The lowest prematurity rates occurred amongst wives in classes I and II where this low rate persisted with all births after the first; in other classes, however, the rate tended to rise with later births reaching a figure of 18 per cent for sixth and subsequent pregnancies.

4 Perinatal Mortality

Perinatal mortality is a measure of mortality at the period of time surrounding birth and includes both stillbirths and early neonatal deaths (i.e. deaths occurring within 1 week of delivery). The perinatal mortality rate is expressed in terms of the number of deaths per 1,000 live births in the corresponding period. Together these two types of death make a considerable contribution to reproductive wastage, and their effects on maternal health frequently produce a vicious circle of maternal morbidity and repeated fetal loss. The stillbirth rate, for women of a particular age, closely parallels the maternal mortality rate, being high for first births, low for second and third but rising steeply thereafter with increasing parity. The early neonatal mortality rate increases uniformly with parity. The heavy contribution of hyperfertile women of low economic status to the wastage of child life at birth has been revealed in a number of studies.[7, 8] The contribution of these mothers to the perinatal mortality rate of urban communities was strikingly demonstrated in a comparative study conducted in Newcastle in 1960. The overall rate of perinatal mortality was 32·7 but the 275 grand multipara showed a rate of 87·3. All of these women belonged to social classes IV and V.[9]

5 Infant Mortality

The infant mortality rate is the number of deaths during the first year of life per 1,000 live births registered in the same period and it clearly reveals the persistence of those factors which have been seen to affect survival even at the intrauterine stage. Indeed the poor economic and social environment, which is only indirectly revealed in perinatal deaths, tends to exacerbate the already reduced life chances of the younger infant in an already large family. The social class and parity correlations of English infant mortality statistics have been well-rehearsed and it is interesting to turn to the United States where, by comparing the vital statistics of white and coloured sections of the population, a similar relationship can be observed (table 22).

TABLE 22. *Birth rates, neonatal and infant mortality rates—USA (rates per 1,000)*

	1940		1950		1965	
	White	Coloured	White	Coloured	White	Coloured
Birth rates	17·9	26·7	23·0	33·3	18·3	27·6
Neonatal mortality	17·2	39·7	19·4	27·5	16·1	25·4
Infant mortality	43·2	73·8	26·8	44·5	21·5	40·3

6 Illegitimacy

Although data on the parity and socio-economic status of the mothers of illegitimate children are not readily available, illegitimate births, taken as a group, portray all those characteristics generally associated with high parity and low social status. Fetal mortality, as shown in table 23, is markedly higher than for legitimate births and the adverse social circumstances and intelligence levels which are usually associated with illegitimate conception place the child at a continuing disadvantage in terms of both physical and intellectual development. Illegitimate births, in England and America, constitute more than 5 per cent of total live births and in both countries the rate is increasing annually. Many illegitimate mothers are teenagers and an unduly large proportion are of low socio-economic status, despite the fact that premarital intercourse is lower amongst these girls than amongst middle-class girls. Obviously lack of contraceptive knowledge is an important factor in illegitimacy and, though it is perhaps unlikely that the majority of potential illegitimate mothers would seek medical advice before the first pregnancy, a second illegitimate pregnancy in the same girl, like a second abortion, reflects adversely on those responsible for her medical welfare.

TABLE 23. *Fetal mortality of illegitimate births in England and Wales— 1964 (rate per 1,000)*

	All infants	Illegitimate infants
Stillbirth rate	16·3	20·2
Early neonatal rate	12·0	17·2
Late neonatal rate	1·8	2·2
Post-neonatal rate	6·1	6·8

7 The Unwanted Child

Illegitimate children are the manifest outcome of a very much larger number of premarital conceptions most of which are legitimized by marriage; they are, by parental decision, unwanted children. Only a quarter of the 60,000 illegitimate children born annually in England and Wales are eventually adopted, a number of them are reared by their mothers but many of the rest become the concern of children's departments and other agencies. Yet the problem of the unwanted child is broader than the problem of illegitimacy. Illegitimate children accounted for less than half of the 30,000 children in care during 1966–7.[10] Of the rest a third were children deserted by their mothers, a fifth were children whose mothers were mentally ill or subnormal and a quarter were the children of parents considered, by the appropriate authority, unfit to be entrusted with their care.

There are many unwanted children who do not find their way into local authority care but who nevertheless become known to social workers because of neglect, cruelty and delinquency. Cruelty to children is an increasing, and abhorrent, social problem. In Britain more than 100,000 become the concern of the National Society for the Prevention of Cruelty to Children each year and, of these, about 10 per cent are the victims of deliberate ill-treatment. In the United States it has been suggested that there are probably one hundred cases for every one seen in hospital, and the problem has become so acute that a number of states are proposing to legislate in order to oblige doctors to notify the authorities when they suspect child neglect or cruelty. Even in households where no such obvious signs of rejection are apparent there may still be a lack of warmth and intimacy or even a lack of positive care which may operate to retard the child's emotional and intellectual development[11] (see also p. 177).

8 The Unplanned Child

Unwanted pregnancies far outnumber unwanted children, and though the personal, emotional and economic burdens they create are less socially apparent, to the individuals concerned they are no less real. On the basis of interviews conducted with 1,500 women attending the maternity booking clinics of two London hospitals it has recently been maintained[12] that one-half of the pregnancies occurring in England are basically unplanned. This confirms the estimate for the US which was proposed on the basis of the findings of the second FGMA study.[13] Family planning, in each of these studies, however, is defined simply in terms of avoiding unwanted pregnancies; very many more couples fail in their timing of a particular conception. Indeed, only a minority of couples can claim to be 'number and spacing planners'; in the GAF study the proportion was a mere 16 per cent.[14]

In advanced industrial societies characterized by high rates of occupational and geographical mobility, where often the wife, as well as the husband, may have a career, and where domestic planning and expenditure must be correlated with (or just allowed to exceed) incremental earnings from a planned career—in these circumstances the advent of an unwanted pregnancy must inevitably add to the anxieties and neuroses which account for so high a proportion of barbiturate consumption in contemporary Britain and America. In societies which have come to expect governmental planning, economic planning and in which individuals plan their domestic outgoings, their careers and their children's educational future the need for planning family growth might be regarded as self-evidently desirable. But whilst governments employ economists and individuals, in other capacities, will take advice of consumers' associations and careers guidance experts, there is a culture lag in the demand for family planning advice. Less than one in five of the London clinic women had received professional contraceptive advice.

9 The Problem Family
In the language of the social worker the problem family is virtually synonymous with the large family. Large families absorb a disproportionate share of remedial social and medical services and they illustrate the inadequacy of the distinction between 'medical' and 'social' in public health provision. A third of London's homeless families are families with three or more children; three-quarters of families with rent arrears in another city were also families of this size. The Ministry of Social Security's recent enquiry[15] into family circumstances revealed that 30 per cent of the 160,000 families with resources below national assistance minima were families with three or more children, and the 1962 National Food Survey showed that families with four or more children had, on average, diets which contained less calcium, protein and calorific intakes than the standards recommended by the British Medical Association. Using a variety of indices, including number of general practitioner consultations, degree of fatigue and number of days'

illness in the previous two weeks, an enquiry amongst 499 urban families in 1965 demonstrated that both maternal and, to a lesser degree, paternal rates of ill-health increased with family size.[16]

The relationship between unregulated, or inadequately controlled, fertility and ill-health is fundamental to a large proportion of the problems of public health, social welfare and educational provision amongst the submerged tenth in contemporary industrial societies. Domiciliary birth control schemes in various cities have shown how the vicious circle of poverty, social inadequacy and hyperfertility can be broken by family planning provision. But the social value of such projects is limited; no spectacular increase in family well-being can result from the prevention of a seventh pregnancy for a woman who already has six children under the age of ten. The long-term aim of preventive medicine must be to ensure that adequate contraceptive advice is available to all women from the outset of their marriages and even before.

10 'Medical' and 'Social' in Medical Practice

The interrelationships between hyperfertility, social inadequacy and ill-health also underline the irrelevance of the traditional distinction between 'medical' and 'social' in preventive medicine. This literally theological distinction originated in the attempt by priests to distinguish between the licit and illicit use of the safe period;[17] it was formally admitted to the vocabulary of medical practice as a political compromise by a Roman Catholic Minister of Health in 1925 and was perpetuated in the Memorandum of 1930.[18]

During the last forty years the distinction has lost whatever meaning it originally had. The dividing line between 'medical' and 'social' is precisely where the community, at any particular time, wishes to draw it. A large number of recent studies of the changing nature of medical practice have stressed the tendency to extend the boundaries of medical care to include whatever may concern the patient's health and well-being. This is not merely regarded as intrinsically desirable but a necessary corrective to the progressive fragmentation of medicine into remote specialisms. *Lancet* has, indeed, suggested that this overall concern with general health should itself be recognized as a specialism and given the name 'holognosiology'![19]

The doctor's reluctance to acknowledge the shift in emphasis is revealed in the use of terms such as 'extended medical grounds', 'medico-

TABLE 24. *Discussion of family planning in different circumstances*

	Circumstances (%)					
Doctor would:	A married woman with mitral stenosis and two children	A married woman with three children and only one bedroom	A married woman with three children and no social or health problems	A married woman of 18 who had just had her first baby	An unmarried woman who had had a baby	A woman just getting married
Introduce subject of family planning himself	90	61	21	38	40	23
Discuss family planning only if asked directly	8	38	74	58	47	74
Not discuss even if asked directly	1	1	4	3	11	2
Sometimes do one sometimes another	1	—	1	1	2	1
Number of doctors* (—100%)	1,383	1,369	1,385	1,384	1,375	1,383

* At each question a small number of doctors, between 0·2 and 1·4 per cent, gave inadequate answers and have been excluded.

social', 'socio-medical' and 'psycho-social'. Indeed, an important part of the function of contemporary psychiatry is that of dressing up social indications and social stresses in quasi-medical terminology.

In the field of family planning the distinction has persisted and is highlighted by a recent enquiry amongst 1,989 doctors in England and Wales.[20] Eighty-two per cent of these said that they spent more time discussing family planning with their patients than they did five years ago, and although 90 per cent felt they should be concerned with the social problems of their families (and fully two-thirds approved of providing family planning clinics for the unmarried) this philosophy was not reflected in the pattern of prescribing. As table 24 shows, there was a greater reluctance to initiate family planning discussion for non-clinical as opposed to strictly clinical indications, though a majority of doctors are obviously sympathetic to patients who themselves raise the question of family planning on other grounds.

THE DOCTOR'S ROLE

All the techniques involved in contraception, and those of terminating a pregnancy in the first three months of gestation, are technically very simple and do not tax a doctor's abilities. It is a disservice to an important subject to pretend otherwise. Often a cap can be fitted and its use taught by nurses or paramedical staff. The prescription of the Pill is generally limited to medical practitioners, but this is more for administrative and legal convenience than for medically defensible reasons. The fitting of IUDs, in suitably screened women, is a sufficiently simple procedure to be carried out by a nurse or midwife under supervision. It is easy to forget that in delivering babies nurses and midwives are given a responsibility which greatly outweighs the majority of practical procedures which doctors undertake. Therapeutic abortion, especially when vacuum aspiration is used, can be done as an outpatient procedure in many cases, although it is always wise to be within easy reach of emergency surgical resources. The degree to which contraceptive procedures are delegated to non-medical people will be very largely determined by the ratio of doctors to patients within a particular country.

The doctor's most important function in the field of contraception is in helping a couple towards a sound choice of method. And, more important, of retaining an awareness of the importance and necessity of adequate contraception in whatever branch of medicine they happen to be working. As in all good medical practice it is imperative to forestall difficulties, and it is bad practice to wait until the couple are overburdened with unnecessary pregnancies and are desperate for help.

THE TECHNIQUES OF FAMILY LIMITATION

The range of contraceptive techniques available to meet the needs of patients has been shown to be wide and varied. It provides for those couples in which one spouse wishes to take the responsibility for contraception and also for those marriages in which birth control is seen as the joint responsibility with husband and wife alternatively adopting their preferred methods. Although the failure rates, amongst the methods described, vary significantly, every method has its convinced adherents because, for most couples, effectiveness is mediated by a range of social and psychological factors which make one method more acceptable than another. Nevertheless, with increasing length of marriage, and especially as the limit of intended family size is approached, reliability becomes a more important consideration and professional advice is likely to be sought. In these circumstances the doctor has a choice of three or four major methods which have tolerable rates of use-effectiveness and the possibility of permanent or quasi-permanent surgical techniques are available to those requiring even greater certainty than is provided by oral and appliance methods. Abortion will remain a necessary adjunct of contraceptive practice and as the public's expectations of effective family planning practice increase it will become correspondingly less defensible to withhold the right of access to termination. In the long term, widespread and unimpeded access to reliable contraceptive methods can only reduce the rate of abortion, especially of criminal abortion.

CONTRACEPTIVE MORTALITY

If contraception confers so many positive medical benefits it also entails certain hazards and, as with all other forms of therapy and surgery, it is important that these should be clearly understood, at least by the practising doctor, and balanced against the consequences of neglect as well as against the dangers attaching to alternative forms of treatment. Coitus, like most good things in life, carries a measurable and inescapable chance of death. Unhappily, the statistics are heavily weighted against the woman, although a not insignificant number of cerebrovascular accidents and coronary thromboses occur to men during sexual intercourse.

The hazards of pregnancy are well understood and until recently reached very high levels. Today, in developed countries, a woman's chances of dying during pregnancy have declined to approximately 1 in 3,000. The dangers attendant on the control of fertility which until recently centred upon the risk of induced, especially criminally induced, abortion are more difficult to estimate. And though deaths from this cause have declined over recent years their contribution to total deaths amongst women is, as has been demonstrated, considerable.

Sterilization, if performed under a general anaesthetic, has always carried a small risk, but as the number of birth control methods increases and as their use becomes more widespread so the possibility of dangerous, even fatal, consequences multiplies. The use of the Pill has now been shown to involve a discernible mortality rate and a number of deaths, together with many more severe infections and perforations, have resulted from the use of the IUD. It is possible, moreover, that further adverse correlations between the use of the Pill and certain diseases will be established. The evidence relating to cervical carcinoma in situ has been reviewed (p. 116). It is relevant to point out that the arithmetic concerning the use of oral contraceptives, especially in the case of carcinoma, is incomplete.[21] It is possible that hormonal agents may protect against certain forms of malignancy although it would be much more difficult to demonstrate that, say, 13 women in a million did not die than that they became corpses; the fact would also be less likely to reach the newspaper headlines.

The difficulties involved in investigating rare side effects due to a contraceptive method and the statistical problems of handling data have already been emphasised. Probably, by the time the effects of the oral contraceptives at present in use have been fully assessed they themselves will have been replaced by newer methods. It is unlikely that young women now taking the Pill will continue to do so until the menopause. Only 2 per cent of pharmacological preparations currently in use were known before the Second World War and contraceptives are now being affected by this pharmacological revolution. Undoubtedly there will be rapid improvement in the present range of contraceptives and a proliferation of new types—which in turn will entail new hazards.

It is necessary to retain a sense of proportion concerning the dangers and side effects of contraceptives. Any aspect of sexual behaviour is, unfortunately, capable of leading to confused and perverse thinking, not least amongst theologians, lawyers and doctors, and some discussion of side effects is therefore justified in both a medical and a social context.

It remains, of course, much more common for a method of family planning to be advised because pregnancy would endanger a woman's life or health than for a method to be contra-indicated because the procedure itself is hazardous. There are no absolute contra-indications to the condom, diaphragm or safe period and they are exceedingly rare for the Pill and IUD. If a man or woman is physically capable of sexual intercourse then sterilization is possible and termination of pregnancy in the first trimester carries less risk than term delivery. From the medical point of view oral contraceptives have aroused most debate, but doctors prescribing the Pill for the first time should remember that it has been in use as a contraceptive for over a decade, that it is currently taken by at least ten million women and that exogenous steroids have been systematically used in much higher dosage for certain gynaecological conditions for over twenty-five years. It is also relevant to recall that many

TABLE 25. *Birth control and maternal mortality rates*

Birth control method (1 million users)	Failure rate	Pregnancies	Women of all ages Annual deaths due to:		
			Pregnancy	Method	Total
Pill	1·0	11,000	3	20	23
IUD	5·0	48,000	12	NK	NK
Condom	10·0	106,000	28	—	28
Coitus interruptus	17·0	170,000	44	—	44
Diaphragm	20·0	200,000	52	—	52
Safe period	23·0	231,000	60	—	60
Douche	31·0	310,000	81	—	81
Therapeutic abortion	—	5,000,000	—	125	125*
Criminal abortion	—	5,000,000	—	2,500	2,500*
Uncontrolled fertility	—	10,000,000	2,600	—	2,600*

* Deaths during reproductive years.

less well-tested and potentially more dangerous drugs are often prescribed more freely than oral contraceptives and some, including tranquillizers, have a more profound effect on human behaviour and raise problems of a type quite unknown in the realm of contraception. All pharmacologically active compounds have some adverse side effects (even aspirin, in normal doses, is not without danger), and it is perhaps surprising that the Pill has not produced more.

It is sometimes suggested that all women using oral contraceptives could be encouraged to use an alternative method but this is unrealistic, unnecessary—and would, even if it were possible, cause avoidable deaths. In fact the most realistic way in which to assess the mortality attributable to oral contraception is to compare a large group of users with similar groups of women who either use some other form of contraception or birth control or, alternatively, choose not to use any form of contraception at all. Table 25 is an attempt to summarize the life chances of ten groups of women, each consisting of a million at the outset, who attempt, respectively, to regulate their childbearing by the use of different contraceptive methods, therapeutic termination or illegal abortion. Normal failure rates, based on the mean of highest and lowest estimates shown in chapter 3, are assumed for the different methods of contraception. For those women relying wholly on abortion or making no attempt to control their fertility, a pregnancy rate of ten per married or cohabiting woman during her reproductive life is adopted, and it is further assumed, in relation to those relying on legal or criminal abortion, that one-half of these pregnancies will end in induced abortion, an estimate which has strong empirical support in the vital statistics of East European countries.

On this basis, oral contraceptives are seen to be both more effective than any other method of birth control and, with the possible exception of the condom, safer than all alternative forms of family limitation. It is difficult to evaluate the death rate for IUDs because not all the background statistics are available, but there is no doubt that they are of the same order as those for oral contraceptives.

The woman who begins taking oral contraceptives has a greater likelihood of being alive one year later than has her sister who chooses to have a baby or to use some less effective method of contraception. A similar conclusion can be reached in another way: supposing some comic opera monarch decreed that every woman in his kingdom—single, widowed, divorced or married, between the ages of 15 and 49 must take oral contraceptives for a year. When the decree expired fewer women would have died in this age-group than during a normal year. On balance, too, the more underdeveloped the society, and the greater the maternal mortality, the greater would be the number of lives saved.

Risks, especially demographic risks, are by their very nature unpredictable and, in the last analysis, the contraceptive Jeremiah may plead that all the accumulated observations on patients and all the animal experiments that might be undertaken would not set his mind at rest. Sir Alan Parkes has pointed out that 'it is always difficult to prove a negative and impossible to do so in advance. In fact we face the dilemma that no women should be kept on the Pill for twenty years until, in fact, a substantial number have been kept on the Pill for twenty years.' The case for prudence is especially strong in medical procedures but there are degrees of prudence. Every new influence which is added to the human environment entails some danger, whether it is a new washing powder, polythene wrapping material, sonic boom or the Pill. Vigilance must be based on sound judgement of all the relevant facts: in the case of the Pill the realities of unwanted children and the population explosion constitute a greater danger than its proven or alleged risks.

However, contraception is not merely a medical prodecure; it is also a social convenience, and if a technique carried a mortality several hundreds of times greater than that now believed to be associated with the Pill its use might still be justified on social if not medical grounds.

TABLE 26. *Deaths/million women England and Wales, 1966*

	Age (years)		
	15–24	25–34	35–44
All causes	427	686	1,705
Accidents, poisoning and violence	148	138	189
(a) Road traffic accidents	87	35	39
(b) Accidental poisoning and drowning	10	18	31
(c) Suicide	30	62	93
Oral contraception	13	13	34

Sexual activity is a powerful driving force for all healthy, mature people and contraceptives need not be judged by the same criteria as broncho-dilators or laxatives. Rather they must be set against the background of their social consequences. Again, to take the specific example of the Pill, the chances of death resulting from its use may be compared with some other risks which are taken daily (table 26). There are a large number of recreational activities which are more dangerous than taking the Pill. In the USA there are over 5,000 boating and swimming fatalities a year and there is ten times the likelihood of a death in the family if father buys an outboard motor boat than if mother uses oral contraceptives. It is probable that the amateur cricketer or footballer (activities which caused twenty-seven deaths in the UK, 1955–8) is more likely to die playing sport at the week-end than his wife is to die from using oral contraceptives.

Almost without exception the consequences of contraception are bene-ficial and contribute significantly to the health and well-being of the community. In contrast, many societies permit drugs and other practices which are of questionable value or are demonstrably harmful. The ill-effects of alcohol and tobacco, which are tolerated for no better reason than that they provide comfort and pleasure, add appreciably to the mortality and morbidity rates of many societies, but they are inade-quately regulated by civil law and social custom and do not fall within the sphere of medical prescription at all. Thirty thousand deaths from lung cancer occur yearly in Britain, the majority due to smoking. By the end of the century more British men will have died from smoking-induced cancer than in two world wars. For every Pill-induced death in Britain there are at least 1,500 cigarette-induced deaths; based on total sales of the two products during 1967 one cigarette is three times as dangerous to life as one Pill. Yet it is one of the paradoxes of modern medicine that the doctor who finds it difficult to persuade a woman to take one Pill a day for three weeks out of four also has difficulty in stopping her husband from smoking 20 cigarettes daily.

All the arguments which have been used in favour of the Pill as opposed to alternative forms of contraception apply with equal validity to the argument for any attempt, by whatever means, to control fertility. Apart from those personal, social and economic advantages which result from family limitation, there is a considerable saving in human life. For the maternal mortality figures shown in table 26 do not represent the limit of reproductive waste; every additional pregnancy resulting from contraceptive failure or non-use makes its incremental contribution to fetal and infant mortality.

FUTURE DEVELOPMENTS IN CONTRACEPTION

Contraceptive practice is not merely a useful surgery or public health technique; it is also an important research frontier on which significant discoveries are likely to be made. In his 1966 Oliver Bird Lecture Sir Solly Zuckerman suggested that reproductive physiology was due for the sort of intellectual breakthrough that has occurred time and time again in physics during the last thirty years, a period in which, he maintained, scarcely anything fundamentally new had been discovered in the physiology of human reproduction. Research in this field is no longer hindered by the sort of attitude which deprived Baker of his bench-space in the 1920s. Nor is it unduly starved of financial support; foundations, unless they are dominated by Catholics (and even the Pope felt obliged to pay lip-service to the value of scientific research), tend to regard fertility control as a desirable cause and there are a number of organizations, some of which are listed in Appendix V, which exist solely or mainly in order to promote investigations in this field.

It is impossible to predict the precise direction of future research, though the lines along which developments are likely to take place during the next decade are reasonably apparent. Much of the history of the development of the Pill was the outcome of a conscious search for an orally effective agent, mainly initiated by Margaret Sanger and executed at the Worcester Foundation, Massachusetts, by Pincus, Chang and their co-workers. There is little doubt that the story could be repeated in other fields and by other centres. There are innumerable links in the complex chain of events making up mammalian reproduction which might be broken and Pincus,[22] Austin and Perry,[23] Jackson[24] and many others[25] have reviewed possible future methods of contraception.

1 Female

(a) HYPOTHALAMUS AND PITUITARY

It might be advantageous to duplicate the effects of the present oral contraceptives in an injectable form. In some cultures, especially developing countries, injections are found to be more acceptable than ingesting tablets. Continuous low doses of progesterone can be achieved by giving intramuscular medroxyprogesterone (Depo Provera). Blood levels are more variable than with daily oral medication and regular menstruation may disappear altogether. One hundred and fifty milligrams given at three-monthly intervals proves an effective contraceptive,[26] but it may take six months or more for fertility to return after the last injection, and if pregnancy occurs before regular cycles have been re-established the progesterone-induced amenorrhea may merge with that of gestation.

In addition to the synthetic steroids now in use, pituitary inhibition or alteration in gonadotrophin release may be achieved by drugs affecting hypothalamic sensitivity or pituitary releasing hormones. Some tranquillizers, for example reserpine, are thought to interfere with the hypothalamic control of releasing hormones and will block ovulation or implantation. Clomiphene is a non-steroidal compound with a variety of interesting actions, one of which may be competition with oestrogen for hypothalamic binding sites. The identification and isolation of pituitary releasing hormones is beginning and may lead to useful results.

The hypothalamus is one of the sites involved in the action of pheromones,[27] that is, substances which are secreted by one individual, often as an odoriferous component of the urine, and which affect the physiology or behaviour of another individual. Pheromones can be used to prolong early pregnancy in the mouse, and although no comparable effect is known in man they demonstrate the complexity of the cerebral control of reproduction.

(b) TARGET ORGANS

It may be possible to block the action of circulatory pituitary gonadotrophins at the peripheral level. Extracts of *Lithospermum ruderal* inactivate gonadotrophins in vitro and some work has been carried out on the immunology of pituitary hormones.

Some of the continuous, low dose contraceptives now being developed and at present subject to clinical trials (preparations that are sometimes christened 'Mini-pills') almost certainly act at the uterine level. Daily dosage with 0·5 mg chlormadinone provides a contraceptive method which is comparable in effectiveness (3·7 pregnancies per HWY over 13,202 cycles)[28] to the IUD but which may have less troublesome side effects. Menstruation occurs against a background of continuous tablet taking and ovulation is only inhibited in a minority of cycles. It is thought that the cervical mucus is hostile to sperm throughout the cycle and it has been demonstrated that sperm are not present in the Fallopian tubes after coitus.[29] Most pregnancies follow tablet omissions. Menstrual irregularities are common but other side effects are rare and lactation is not altered in any way.

(c) POST-COITAL PILLS

The balance of pituitary and ovarian hormones remains of the utmost importance after ovulation and unless a specific sequence of progesterone and oestrogen occurs, transportation and implantation of the fertilized egg cannot take place. In rats stress, or lactation following a previous pregnancy, interferes with implantation and it has been noted (chapter 9) that the combination preparations of oral contraceptives may act in this way. Oestrogens prevent implantation when given in high doses for three days after mating in the rabbit or for six days after mid-cycle mating in the macaque monkey. Preliminary trials in women have been promising and no pregnancies occurred in over one hundred women exposed to mid-cycle unprotected intercourse when they were given 25 to 50 mg stilboestrol or 0·5 to 2 mg ethynyl oestradiol daily for five days after the coitus.[30] Nausea commonly accompanies these high doses of oestrogen but an effective post-coital preparation would have a limited but useful place in fertility control. A variety of anti-oestrogens is known which inhibits implantation in rodents. It appears to have little or no effect in primates but it is possible that an anti-implantation compound could be developed for routine use as a once-a-month pill.

(d) ABORTIFACIENTS

The steroid hormones responsible for the maintenance of pregnancy during the first three months of human gestation are produced by the corpus luteum. In some species, such as the sheep and pig, a luteolytic hormone produced by the endometrium has been demonstrated, which destroys the corpus luteum unless implantation and early development have taken place.[31] As the control of corpus luteum regression in the human situation is explored it may present a suitable site for the control of fertility. In Sweden Ferrosavy G 103, bis-(p-acetoxyphenyl)-2-methyl cyclohexylidenemethane, has been proved a partially effective abortifacient in women and its action is probably that of interfering with the luteal synthesis of progesterone.[32] In England, Kirby has shown that antilymphocytic sera causes abortion in laboratory rodents, possibly because it contains a component causing corpus luteum destruction.

There is no doubt that an abortifacient pill or injection would be exceedingly useful and would be widely used. The clinical effects of spontaneous abortion at five or six weeks are relatively mild and subsequent dilatation and curettage, while necessary in some cases, might not have to be very widely used. There are also a number of embryotrophin agents that would cause abortion; only in these cases the opportunity for surgical termination would have to be at hand in case of teratological effects such as are known to occur with aminopterin.

2   Male

The range of female contraceptives is now much wider and more sophisticated than those available to men, and it is paradoxical that male techniques—limited to the centuries-old methods of coitus interruptus and the condom—remain the most widely used and have contributed most to the decline in the birth rate of developed nations. No degree of ingenuity will make any fundamental difference to the one reversible method of mechanical contraception but there is a great need to give the sexes some equality of opportunity in the choice of oral or injectable methods.

(a) CHEMICAL

The number of possible sites for interrupting fertility is almost as large in the male as in the female. Sperm production and maturation is a complex process. Many compounds are known to reduce sperm production and one of the bis-(dichloroacetyl)-diamines has been used on men with some success. A difficulty encountered with male oral contraception is that the sperm produced in the seminiferous tubules take two to three months to reach the ejaculate. The bis-(dichloroacetyl)-diamine,

$Cl_2CHCONH (CH_2)_8 NOCOCHCl_2$ (Win 18446), tried on men led to low sperm counts after 50 days and complete azoospermia after 80 days. Conversely, fertility took 100 days to be fully restored. The drug was tested (125–1,000 mg daily) on twenty-seven volunteers in American penitentiaries[33] and appeared to be successful until it was found to cause acute distress (rather like the effect of Antabuse) 10 to 20 min after taking alcohol. It is to be hoped that adequate chemical control of male fertility will be achieved but it must be remembered that, in addition to the delay factor, the twin biological problems of selectively blocking spermatogenesis without involving other dividing cells, such as the bone marrow, and of avoiding possible teratological effects are formidable. Sperm taken from the testes or vas deferens will not fertilize an egg, and in most species sperm have to be exposed to a uterine environment in order to become fully 'capacitated' and it may prove possible to halt the maturation of sperm without interfering with their production. For example, the mono-esters of methanesulphonic acid are effective in this way.[34]

Male fertility is very susceptible to changes in gonadotrophins and steroid hormones although it is difficult to produce infertility without reducing libido.

(b) IMMUNOLOGICAL

The possibility of obtaining immunization against pregnancy is an attractively simple one and it has a long and hopeful history. It was first explored by Landsteiner in 1899[35] and in 1932 Baskin took out a US patent in immunological contraception. In theory the method is applicable to either sex but more work has been done on the male side, partly because some types of pathological infertility have an immunological basis. Aspermatogenesis can be produced in male animals by immunization techniques, but so far they have involved the use of Freund's adjuvant which produces a very marked local reaction and there is no immediate prospect of applying the technique to human reproduction. Given an effective technique it might still be difficult to make it reversible.

3 Sociological

The future advancement of contraceptive practice will depend no less on the findings of sociology than on the discoveries of the biological sciences. A 'perfect' method of birth control, universally acceptable in all situations, independent of the volitional decisions of individuals and without side effects or hazards of any kind, is not remotely within sight; and when it becomes available it will doubtless raise a new set of sociological issues. In the meantime we are stuck with a range of techniques of varying efficacy whose acceptability is more closely related to cultural factors than to their theoretical efficiency.

Sociological research during the last thirty years has contributed significantly to our understanding of some of the social influences affecting reproductive behaviour. These have been referred to in the foregoing chapters, but there remain important gaps in our knowledge. We lack, for example, an objective evaluation of the acceptability, reliability and use-effectiveness of even the major techniques in broadly comparable cultural situations. Nor do we know what factors affect the choice of method, or the degree of knowledge upon which the choice is made, in western societies; still less do we know the reasons for its subsequent rejection for an alternative technique.

There is no completely satisfactory explanation for the problem of differential fertility in industrial countries. The apparent irrelevance of family planning amongst the lowest socio-economic groups is difficult to reconcile with the unquestionable success of domiciliary schemes in which birth control has been readily accepted by these same couples. But if such sections of the population are to be given the maximum help which modern family planning affords it is necessary to be able to predict the type of couple who will become the hyperfertile parents of the next generation.

The recent apparent trend towards larger families amongst the better-off sections of advanced societies has been the subject of much comment, theorizing and speculation: the factors responsible for this reversal of the demographic trends of the last sixty years remain unexplored. At an even more general level we are largely ignorant of the factors responsible for decisions on desired family size or of the circumstances in which these may be revised. Yet this is the most important factor contributing to population growth in advanced societies. Completed families of 2·5 children in Britain and America would result in a stabilizing of population growth; completed families of 3·5 children would result in a doubling of the population in 40 years. Yet we have no knowledge of the factors which may induce the present generation of married couples to choose between these rather narrow alternatives.

The GAF and FGMA studies in America and the PIC survey in

Britain have done much to enlarge our knowledge of recent and contemporary contraceptive practice, but it has been pointed out that the current trend is away from this sort of 'large scale investigation involving the multivariate analysis of many conflicting factors and their effects. It is believed that smaller samples, investigated in greater depth, should prove more useful. Such inquiries would involve not only information about family-building in the past but also statements of intention as to

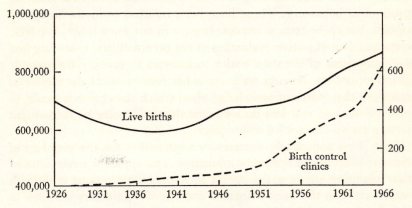

Fig. 39. Annual births and FPA clinics, England and Wales. 1926–66.

the future: only in this way can a full picture of the current situation be obtained.'[36] The experience gained during the large-scale surveys of the last twenty years has been condensed into a set of recommendations[37] for inclusion in national censuses which will, if adopted, obviate the need for independent enquiries in the future.

There remains a great deal to be discovered about the history of birth control in the advanced societies. In particular, the precise function of the voluntary clinic movement has never been fully assessed. Indeed, a mischievous statistician could argue, on the basis of the data shown in figure 39, that the effect of the clinics on the English birth rate was a negative one. Certainly, the contribution of the clinics to family limitation must be assessed much more in terms of their contribution to educating public and governmental opinion than in their practical activities.

In overseas family planning programmes the need for sociological and statistical evaluation and assessment of action programmes is accepted. All programmes and innovations initiated by the IPPF are now preceded by 'Knowledge, Attitude and Practice' studies, the accumulated results of which will be invaluable to future activities.[38] Motivation and communications research in underdeveloped countries is a further field of enquiry which is only just beginning to be developed.

There can be few other fields of scientific study which offer so many opportunities for original and significant research. If Laski, writing in 1932, was premature in his judgement that contraceptive study had undergone the transition from the stage of enthusiasm to the stage of science, developments in the intervening period have at least furnished an unchallengeable scientific basis from which the work of the next decade can proceed. Even the case against contraception must now be argued from fact rather than from prejudice; indeed, the scientists are now apparently so secure in their convictions and knowledge that they feel able to adopt the invective which has so long been the monopoly of their opponents. It was a leading scientific journal which, apropos of the 1968 Papal Encyclical, declared: 'Bigotry, pedantry and fanaticism can kill, maim, and agonise those upon whom they are visited just as surely as bombs, pogroms and the gas chamber. Pope Paul VI has now gently joined the company of tyrants, but the damage he has done may well outclass and outlast that of all earlier oppressors.'[39]

Appendix I IPPF AGREED TEST FOR TOTAL SPERMICIDAL POWER (1965)

Minimal Requirements for Semen to be Used for Testing

Sample age: Not more than 4 hours old.

Density: 50 million/ml.

Motility: 40 to 50 per cent of the sperms should show rapid forward motion when examined with a fresh mount at 35 to 37 °C.

Viscosity: Properly liquefied semen, not 'stringy' when run out of a pipette, and appearing homogeneous to the naked eye.

Specimens must not be collected in a rubber or latex sheath or condom and should be kept tightly stoppered in a tube at room temperature before being tested.

Apparatus Required

0·9 per cent saline solution.

Magnetic mixer (magnet of synchronous motor or similar device).

Stainless-steel lockwasher (1·2 × 0·2 cm) or other suitable magnetic stirrer.

Glass or polyethylene-coated magnetic stirrer (2·5 × 0·7 cm).

Test tubes, 85 × 15 mm, thick-walled.

Pipettes as required.

Stopclock.

Microscope, slides, etc.

Incubator or waterbath (at 35 to 37 °C).

Control Test for Effect of Dilution and Magnetic Mixing

The following control test should be done on each specimen of semen just before it is used for the spermicidal tests. If the semen is in use for more than 2 hours the control test should be repeated.

Procedure

1 Bring all materials to 35 to 37 °C, using incubator or waterbath.

2 Pipette 0·2 ml of semen into test tube, taking care that no semen splashes up the sides of the tube.

3 Add lockwasher or other magnetic stirrer, insert tube in field of magnetic mixer. Check that mixer is working.

4 Add 1·0 ml of saline, simultaneously starting mixer and timer. This is zero time.
5 Let mix for 10 s. Place a drop on a plain slide, cover with cover-slip, and put on microscope stage.
6 At 40 s (i.e. 30 s after end of mixing) rapidly examine 5 fields with low power (100 to 150 ×), followed by 5 fields with high power (400 to 600 ×).
7 If activity in the dilution is not satisfactory in terms of the original assessment, the sample of semen must be discarded.
8 Add 1·0 ml of buffered glucose solution, mix, and re-examine for sperm activity after 30 min at 37 °C.

The Test Proper

Dilutions of spermicidal products should be made up freshly with a 0·9 per cent NaCl solution, just before the test is to be done. 1·0 g of the product is weighed into a 50 ml beaker and 11·0 ml of normal saline are added (1 : 11 or 1 in 12 solution); this solution is kept at 35 to 37 °C for 15 min. After this period, the spermicidal solution is mixed for 15 min at 35 to 37 °C if possible, otherwise at room temperature (22 to 25 °C), using a glass or polyethylene-coated magnetic stirrer. Following this mixing the solution is allowed to stand at 35 to 37 °C for 30 min. Immediately before each test the spermicidal solution is stirred 20 times, using a glass rod.

The pH of the solution is recorded, using a universal indicator solution or pH meter, but not indicator papers. In the case of foaming tablets one reading is taken while foaming is in progress and a second when foam is completely exhausted.

Procedure

1 Bring all material to 35 to 37 °C, using incubator or waterbath.
2 Place 0·2 ml of warm semen in test tube, taking care that no semen splashes up the sides of the test tube, since this might cause a false fail.
3 Add lockwasher or other magnetic stirrer, insert tube in field of magnetic mixer. Check that mixer is working.
4 Add 1·0 ml of the warm spermicidal solution prepared as above, simultaneously starting mixer and timer. This is zero time.
5 Let mix for 10 s. Place a drop on a plain slide, cover with cover-slip, and put on microscope stage.
6 At 40 s examine 5 fields rapidly with low power (100 to 150 ×). If no motility is observed confirm by examining at least 5 fields under high power (400 to 600 ×). If even a single sperm shows any sign of life 'jerking or swimming' score 'fail'. If no sperms show any sign of life, score 'preliminary pass'.
7 If no active sperms are found, add 1·0 ml of buffered glucose solution to the tube containing the semen–spermicide mixture. Stir well with glass rod or mix well by drawing the fluid into pipette and running out 3 times. Place in incubator for about 30 min and re-examine as above. If still no active sperms are seen, score 'final pass'.

Result

It is suggested that the product reaches a desirable level of spermicidal activity provided 1·0 ml of a 1:11 solution kills all sperms in 0·2 ml of semen under the conditions of the test as described above. Each product should be tested against semen from 3 different individuals; if all sperms are killed in these 3 samples then the product is accepted. If it fails to do this in 2 out of 3 or in all 3 then it is regarded as unacceptable. If it fails with 1 semen sample then the whole test is repeated using 3 different semen samples, and only if it kills all sperms in all of these new semen samples can it be regarded as having reached a desirable level of spermicidal activity; in other words, only 1 fail is permitted out of 6 tests.

Appendix II THE BRITISH STANDARDS INSTITUTION TESTS FOR RUBBER CONDOMS

A Test for Holes

1 Fit the specimen on the end of a suitable mount of about 1¾in. (44·5 mm) diameter. Suitable equipment is illustrated.

2 Ensure that the outer surface of the specimen is in a dry state. Then add 300 ml of water, taking measures to ensure that air is expelled, and suspend freely for not less than 3 min.

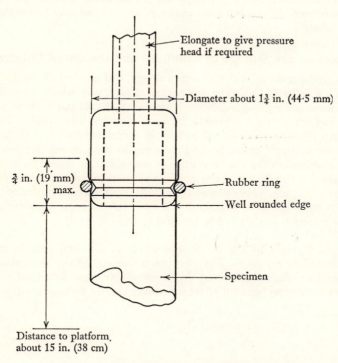

Fig. 40. Equipment for testing rubber condoms.

267

3 Test for leakage of water through the walls of the article by wrapping round it a sheet of dry filter paper which shall on removal be inspected for signs of leakage.

Condoms which have been treated with lubricants during manufacture may be visually examined for water leakage.

B Bursting Strength Test for Condoms

1 For specimens tested before ageing. (a) Fit the specimen on the end of a suitable mount of about $1\frac{3}{4}$ in. (44·5 mm) diameter, which is situated about 15 in. (38 cm) above a platform upon which the lower part of the specimen undergoing test may rest when it is filled with water. Suitable equipment is illustrated. (b) Add 3 l. of water to the specimen. If necessary, an excess pressure head may be employed to initiate inflation.

2 For specimens tested after ageing. (a) Accelerated ageing of the specimen shall be undertaken by the air oven method in accordance with BS 903, Part A 19, at a temperature of 70 °C for 168 hours (7 days), after which the specimen shall be taken from the oven and allowed to cool for not less than 12 hours. (b) Fit the specimen on the end of a suitable mount of about $1\frac{3}{4}$ in. (44·5 mm) diameter. Suitable equipment is illustrated. (c) Add 2 l. of water to the specimen. If necessary, an excess pressure head may be employed to initiate inflation.

C Notes on the Storage of Condoms and the use of Lubricants

Storage. Rubber tends to deteriorate with age, and particularly in the case of thin-walled articles. Condoms are packaged in a way which normally will protect them during storage. Nonetheless, they should not be kept in stock longer than is necessary, especially in warm climates. The articles should be stored in a cool place and should be kept in containers such that the contents will not be subjected to mechanical damage. As soon as any condom shows any deterioration of the characteristics of the rubber, it should be destroyed.

The articles should not at any time be allowed to come into contact with oil-based antiseptic, phenols and their derivatives, petroleum-based grease, petroleum spirit, paraffin (kerosene) and other related organic products, since all these materials are extremely harmful to rubber.

Lubricants. Because of the deleterious effect of oil- and petroleum-based grease, including petroleum jelly, these materials should not be used to lubricate condoms made of rubber. A water-soluble base lubricant or other lubricant having no harmful effect on rubber should be employed.

Appendix III LIST OF CONTRACEPTIVE PRODUCTS AVAILABLE IN ENGLAND AND THE UNITED STATES

There are many thousands of different contraceptive products, including one hundred brands of oral contraceptive; sometimes the same product is sold under different names in different countries. The following is a list of the principle manufacturers together with those of their products that are available, and appear to be well established, in the United Kingdom or America.

1 UNITED KINGDOM

Product	Name of manufacturer or supplier	Testing agency
IUDs		
Birnberg Bow	Schueler & Company	PC
Gräfenberg Ring	John Bell & Croyden	PC
Gynekoil	Ortho Pharmaceutical	PC
Hall Stone Ring	Allen & Hanbury	CIFC
Lippes Loop	Ortho Pharmaceutical	PC
Saf-T-Coil	London Rubber Industries	PC
ORALS		
Anovlar	Schering A.G.	CIFC
Anovlar-21	Schering A.G.	CIFC
Conovid	G. D. Searle	CIFC
Enavid	G. D. Searle	FPA
Feminor Sequential	London Rubber Industries	
Gynovlar	Schering A.G.	CIFC
Lyndiol	Organon Laboratories	CIFC
Lyndiol 2·5	Organon Laboratories	CIFC
Minovlar	Schering A.G.	
Norinyl-L	Syntex Laboratories	DC
Norinyl-1	Syntex Laboratories	DC
Norlestrin	Parke, Davis	FPA
Orthonovin	Ortho Pharmaceutical	FPA

Product	Name of manufacturer or supplier	Testing agency
Ovulen	G. D. Searle	CIFC
Previson	Roussel Pharmaceuticals	CIFC
*Serial-28	British Drug Houses	DC
*Volidan	British Drug Houses	CIFC

* Available in Ireland

CAPS, DIAPHRAGMS

CBC Racial Cap	Lamberts (Dalston)	FPA
Clinocap	Lamberts (Dalston)	FPA
Dumas Cap	Lamberts (Dalston)	FPA
Durex Check Pessary	London Rubber Industries	FPA
Durex Coil Spring Diaphragms	London Rubber Industries	FPA
Durex Flat Spring Diaphragms	London Rubber Industries	FPA
Lam Butt Cap Pessary	Lamberts (Dalston)	FPA
Lam Butt Diaphragm	Lamberts (Dalston)	FPA
Ortho Diaphragm	Ortho Pharmaceutical	FPA
Plastic Dumas Cap	Lamberts (Dalston)	FPA
Vimule Pessary	Lamberts (Dalston)	FPA

CONDOMS

Beatalls Veribest Gold Pack	London Rubber Industries	CA
CBC Lubricated	London Rubber Industries	CA
Durapac	London Rubber Industries	CA
Durex Coral Supertrans	London Rubber Industries	CA
Durex Gossamer	London Rubber Industries	CA
Durex Nu-Pack	London Rubber Industries	CA
Durex Paragon (several types)	London Rubber Industries	CA
Durex Protectives	London Rubber Industries	CA
Durex Washable Sheaths	London Rubber Industries	CA
Lam Butt Coral Superfine	Lamberts (Dalston)	CA
Ona Coral Supertrans	London Rubber Industries	CA
Ona Protectives	London Rubber Industries	CA
Premex Coral Superfine	Premier Laboratories	CA
Prevax	London Rubber Industries	CA
Transparent Paragon	London Rubber Industries	CA
Transyl	London Rubber Industries	CA
Velsan	London Rubber Industries	CA

SPERMICIDES

Antemin Cream	Coates & Cooper	IPPF
Arloid Foam Tablets	Lloyds Surgical Dept.	IPPF
Arloid Gel Suppositories	Lloyds Surgical Dept.	IPPF
Bircon Foaming Tablets	London Rubber Industries	IPPF

Product	Name of manufacturer or supplier	Testing agency
Bymeston Foam Tablets	Lamberts (Dalston)	IPPF
Delfen Cream	Ortho Pharmaceutical	IPPF
Delfen Vaginal Foam	Ortho Pharmaceutical	IPPF
Dura Gel	London Rubber Industries	IPPF
Efpa Gel	Ortho Pharmaceutical	IPPF
Emko Vaginal Foam	Emko	CA
GP Jelly	Gilmont Products	IPPF
GP Ointment	Gilmont Products	IPPF
GP Soluble Pessaries	Gilmont Products	IPPF
Genexol Cream	W. J. Rendell	IPPF
Gynomin	Coates & Cooper	IPPF
Mallpass Foam Tablets	Mallpass (Pharmaceuticals)	IPPF
Ortho Creme	Ortho Pharmaceutical	IPPF
Ortho-Gynol Jelly	Ortho Pharmaceutical	IPPF
Ortho-forms	Ortho Pharmaceutical	IPPF
Parvol	British Drug Houses	IPPF
Preceptin Gel	Ortho Pharmaceutical	MSRB
Rendells	W. J. Rendell	IPPF
Staycept	Stayne Laboratories	IPPF
Staycept Jelly	Stayne Laboratories	IPPF
Staycept Vaginal Suppositories	Stayne Laboratories	IPPF
Volfam Cream	Aries	IPPF
Volfam Foam Tablets	Aries	IPPF
Volpar Gels	British Drug Houses	IPPF
Volpar Paste	British Drug Houses	IPPF
Volpar Foam Tablets	British Drug Houses	IPPF

2 UNITED STATES

IUDs

Birnberg Bow	Schueler	PC
Comet	Skye-Ray Medical Supply	
Gynekoil	Ortho Pharmaceutical	PC
Hall Stone Ring	Goshen Instrument	
Lippes Loop	Ortho Pharmaceutical	PC
Majzlin Spring	Anka Research	
Saf-T-Coil	Julius Schmid	

ORALS

C-Quens	Eli Lilly	FDA
Enovid	G. D. Searle	FDA
Enovid-E	G. D. Searle	FDA

Product	Name of manufacturer or supplier	Testing agency
Norinyl-L	Syntex	FDA
Norinyl-1	Syntex	FDA
Norlestrin	Parke, Davis	FDA
Ovulen	G. D. Searle	FDA
Oracon	Mead Johnson	FDA
Orthonovin	Ortho Pharmaceutical	FDA
Orthonovin-SQ	Ortho Pharmaceutical	FDA
Provest	Upjohn	FDA

CAPS, DIAPHRAGMS

Bendex Diaphragms	Julius Schmid
Coil Spring Diaphragms	Julius Schmid
Koroflex Diaphragms	Holland Rantos
Koromex Diaphragms	Holland Rantos
Mensinga Diaphragms	Holland Rantos
Milex Cervical Caps	Milex Products
Milex Diaphragms	Milex Products
Ortho Cervical caps	Ortho Pharmaceutical
Ortho Diaphragms	Ortho Pharmaceutical

CONDOMS

Circle	Circle Rubber Co.
Dean	Dean Rubber Manufacturing
Many Brands	Julius Schmid
Many Brands	Killashun International
Many Brands	L. E. Shunk Latex Products
Many Brands	Lorica
Many Brands	Young's Rubber

SPERMICIDES

Bilco Jelly	Veritas Products	MSRB
Certane Jelly	Vogarell Products	MSRB
Certane Cream	Vogarell Products	MSRB
Colagyn Jel	The Smith Laboratory	MSRB
Cooper Creme	Whittakers Laboratories	IPPF
Cooper Creme Gel	Whittakers Laboratories	IPPF
Creemoz Vaginal Creme	Larre Laboratories	IPPF
Delfen Cream	Ortho Pharmaceutical	IPPF
Delfen Vaginal Foam	Ortho Pharmaceutical	IPPF
Durafoam Powder with Sponge	Durex Products	IPPF
Durafoam Liquid with Sponge	Durex Products	IPPF
Durafoam Tablets	Durex Products	IPPF
Emko Vaginal Foam	Emko	IPPF
Esta Gel	Esta Medical Laboratories	IPPF

Product	Name of manufacturer or supplier	Testing agency
Immolin Cream-Jel	Julius Schmid	IPPF
Jellak Jelly	Larre Laboratories	IPPF
Kemi Cream	Kemi Products	MSRB
Kemi Jelly	Kemi Products	MSRB
Koromex A Jelly	Holland Rantos	IPPF
Koromex Cream	Holland Rantos	IPPF
Koromex Jelly	Holland Rantos	IPPF
Lactikol Creme	Durex Products	IPPF
Lactikol Jelly	Durex Products	IPPF
Lanesta Gel	Esta Medical Laboratories	IPPF
Lantan Jelly	Esta Medical Laboratories	IPPF
L.A.L. Jelly	Veritas Products	MSRB
Lorocol Jelly	Peck & Sterba Division	IPPF
Lorocol D Jelly	Peck & Sterba Division	IPPF
Lorophyn Jelly	Eaton Laboratories	IPPF
Lorophyn Suppositories	Eaton Laboratories	IPPF
Marvosan Creme	Veritas Products	MSRB
Marvosan Jelly	Veritas Products	MSRB
Milex Crescent Creme	Milex Products	MSRB
Milex Crescent Jelly	Milex Products	MSRB
Ortho Creme	Ortho Pharmaceutical	IPPF
Ortho-Gynol Jelly	Ortho Pharmaceutical	IPPF
Preceptin Gel	Ortho Pharmaceutical	MSRB
Ramses Jelly	Julius Schmid	IPPF
Veritas Kreme	Veritas Products	MSRB
Verithol	Veritas Products	MSRB
Zeptabs	Larre Laboratories	IPPF

CA	Consumers Association
CIFC	Council for the Investigation of Fertility Control
DC	Dunlop Committee on the Safety of Drugs
FDA	Food and Drug Administration
FPA	Family Planning Association
IPPF	International Planned Parenthood Federation
MSRB	Margaret Sanger Research Bureau
PC	Population Council

The listing of a product does not necessarily imply that it has passed the tests of the agency concerned.

Appendix IV

SUGGESTED REQUIREMENTS FOR THE INSERTION OF INTRAUTERINE CONTRACEPTIVE DEVICES

Speculum, bivalve.
Vosellum (27 cm).
Uterine sounds, curved.
Hegar dilators, sizes 3, 4, 5.
Sponge forceps (27 cm).
Cheatle forceps.
Artery forceps.
Scissors, curved.

Kidney dishes and lids.
Lotion bowls.
Cottonwool (absorbent).
Sterilizing solution.
Gloves (sterilized rubber or sterilized disposable).
Sanitary towels.

RESUSCITATION EQUIPMENT

Double-ended airway.
Mouth gag.
Ampoules of adrenaline.

Disposable, pre-sterilized syringes and needles.

Appendix V

ORGANIZATIONS SPECIALIZING IN THE FIELD OF CONCEPTION CONTROL

Eugenics Society,
69 Eccleston Square,
London S.W.1

Supports research projects over a wide field in the biological and social sciences including clinical and sociological aspects of family planning

Family Planning Association,
27–35 Mortimer Street,
London W.C.1

Administers 700 clinics in England and Wales; publishes quarterly journal 'Family Planning'

Ford Foundation,
320 East 43rd Street,
New York

Provides financial support to US universities specializing in demography, family planning training and research; aids overseas schemes for fertility control

Hugh Moore Fund,
60 East 42nd Street,
New York

Supports family planning organizations and research projects

International Planned Parenthood
 Federation,
18–20 Lower Regent Street,
London S.W.1

Co-ordinates activities of 54 member countries; maintains library and information service; organizes international conferences; sponsors research; publishes range of clinical and sociological literature

The Lalor Foundation,
Wilmington,
Delaware

Supports research on all aspects of reproduction but especially those which, because of public prejudice, are unlikely to attract support elsewhere

Milbank Memorial Fund,
40 Wall Street,
New York

Supports research fellowships in public health, preventive medicine and demography. Publishes journal 'Milbank Memorial Fund Quarterly'

National Committee on Maternal
 Health,
2 East 103rd Street,
New York

Conducts research and publishes occasional papers, including periodical bibliographies on fertility control, available gratis to students and clinicians

Pathfinder Fund, 1575 Tremont Street, Boston	*Sponsors field programmes in fertility control; provides free contraceptive supplies for use in underdeveloped countries*
Planned Parenthood Federation of America, 515 Madison Avenue, New York	*Parent organization of 154 state federations; sponsors educational and promotional activities*
Population Council, 245 Park Avenue, New York	*Performs and supports research on contraceptive methods; sponsors educational programmes and films; publishes 'Studies in Family Planning'*
Rockefeller Foundation, 111 West 50th Street, New York	*Sponsors and supports research on population and fertility control*
Sociological Research Foundation, 50 Pall Mall, London s.w.1	*Constituted by trust deed to sponsor and support research on fertility control*
Victor Fund, 1730 K Street, Washington	*Fund-raising organization for work of IPPF*
World Health Organization, Geneva, Switzerland	*Sponsors and finances research on the biology of reproduction*

References

Chapter 1

1 H. Sigerist, *History of Medicine*, Vol. 1 (New York, 1950).
2 O. Temkin, *Soranus' Gynaecology* (Baltimore, 1956).
3 [G. Drysdale], *Physical, Sexual and Natural Religion* (London, 1854). *The Elements of Social Science* (London, 1937).
4 B. & P. Russell, *The Amberley Papers* (London, 1937).
5 C. H. F. Routh in *Med. Press Circ.* (1878).
6 J. A. Banks, *Prosperity and Parenthood* (London, 1954).
7 *Lancet*, 11 August 1917.
8 F. Watson, *Dawson of Penn* (London, 1950).
9 Sir J. Marchant (ed.), *Medical Views on Birth Control* (London, 1926).
10 A. J. Cronin, *The Citadel* (London, 1937).
11 N. E. & V. C. Himes, *Hosp. Soc. Serv.* **19** (1929); L. S. Florence, *Birth Control on Trial* (London, 1930).
12 E. Charles, *The Practice of Birth Control* (London, 1932).
13 H. M. Carlton & H. Florey, *J. Obstet. Gynaec. Br. Emp.* **38** (1931).
14 *The Artificial Production of Sterility by the Use of Spermatoxins*. Report to the BCIC by Dr C. F. Cosin (1931).
15 H. M. Carlton & H. J. Phelps, *J. Obstet. Gynaec. Br. Emp.* **40** (1933).
16 B. P. Wiesner in *International Medical Group for the Investigation of Birth Control*. First report (ed. Blacker) (1928).
17 S. Zuckerman, *J. Physiol.* **99** (1937).
18 J. R. Baker, *The Chemical Control of Conception* (London, 1935).
19 Personal communication from Dr J. R. Baker, 2 September 1962.
20 SPBCC, Annual Report (1927–8).
21 FPA *Speakers' Notes* (1962).
22 M. Sanger, *My Fight for Birth Control* (New York and London, 1932).
23 P. Fryer, *The Birth Controllers* (London, 1965).
24 A. M. Stone & N. E. Himes, *Practical Birth Control Methods* (New York, 1938).
25 A. Guttmacher, preface to 1963 edition of N. E. Himes, *Medical History of Contraception* (New York, 1963).
26 A. M. Ward, *J. Biosoc. Sci.* **1** (1969).

Chapter 2

1 F. Lorimer, *Culture and Human Fertility* (UNESCO, Paris, 1954).
2 T. R. Malthus, *An Essay on the Principles of Population* (1798).

3 Royal Commission on Population, *Report* (1949).
4 J. A. Banks, *Prosperity and Parenthood* (London, 1957).
5 A. C. Benson & Viscount Esher, *The Letters of Queen Victoria 1837–1861* (London, 1907).
6 J. W. Innes, *Class Fertility Trends in England and Wales 1876–1934* (London, 1938).
7 J. A. & O. Banks, *Popul. Stud.* **8** (1954).
8 H. B. Bonner, *Charles Bradlaugh: A Record of His Life and Work* (London, 1908).
9 D. V. Glass, *Population Policies and Movements in Europe* (London, 1940).
10 J. Peel, *Popul. Stud.* **18** (1962).
11 E. Lewis-Faning, *Family Limitation and its Influence on Human Fertility during the Past Fifty Years* (London, 1949).
12 R. Freedman in *Research in Family Planning* (ed. Kiser) (Princeton, 1961).
13 P. K. Whelpton, *Social and Psychological Factors Affecting Fertility* (New York, 1946–58).
14 G. Rowntree & R. Pierce, *Popul. Stud.* **16** (1961).
15 P. K. Whelpton *et al.*, *Fertility and Family Planning in the United States* (Princeton, 1966).
16 C. F. Westoff, *Studies in Family Planning*, **17** (1967).
17 J. Kincaid, *Br. Med. J.* **2** (1965).
18 L. Rainwater, *And the Poor Get Children* (Chicago, 1960).
19 M. Peberdy in *Biological Aspects of Social Problems* (eds. Meade and Parkes) (Edinburgh, 1965).
20 H. F. Dorn, *The Population Dilemma* (ed. Hauser) (Englewood Cliffs, 1963).
21 J. Hajnal in *Population in History* (ed. Glass and Eversley) (London, 1965).
22 P. R. Cox, *Eugen. Rev.* **56** (1964).

Chapter 3

1 C. I. B. Voge, *Mfg. Chem.* (1933).
2 C. I. B. Voge, *The Chemistry and Physics of Contraception* (London, 1933).
3 J. R. Baker, R. M. Ranson & J. Tynen, *Camb. J. Hyg.* **37** (1937).
4 IPPF, *Medical Handbook on Contraception* (London, 1965).
5 W. H. Masters & V. E. Johnson, *Human Sexual Response* (London, 1966).
6 C. F. Westoff, R. G. Potter & P. C. Sagi, *The Third Child* (Princeton, 1963).
7 M. Stopes, *The First Five Thousand* (London, 1925).
8 N. Haire, *Practitioner*, **111** (1923).
9 R. Pearl, *Hum. Biol.* **4** (1932).
10 L. Henry, *Eugen. Q.* **8** (1961).
11 R. G. Potter & P. C. Sagi in *Research in Family Planning* (ed. Kiser) (Princeton, 1961).
12 M. Peberdy in *Biological Aspects of Social Problems* (eds. Meade and Parkes) (Edinburgh, 1965).

Chapter 4

1 D. V. Glass, *Population Policies and Movements in Europe* (London, 1940).
2 E. Lewis-Faning, *Family Limitation and its Influence on Human Fertility during the Past Fifty Years* (London, 1949).
3 G. Rowntree & R. Pierce, *Popul. Stud.* (1961).
4 R. Freedman, P. K. Whelpton & A. A. Campbell, *Family Planning, Sterility and Population Growth* (New York, 1959).
5 N. Himes, *Medical History of Contraception* (London, 1936 and 1963).
6 J. M. Stycos & K. W. Back, *The Family and Population Control* (North Carolina, 1955).
7 M. Potts, *Eugen. Rev.* **60** (1967).
8 S. Poti, C. R. Malaker & B. Chakraborti, *Proceedings of the Sixth International Conference on Planned Parenthood* (London, 1959).
9 J. N. Sinher, *Second All India Conference on Family Planning* (Bombay, 1955).
10 L. S. Florence, *Progress Report on Birth Control* (London, 1956).
11 C. F. Westoff in *Social and Psychological Factors Affecting Fertility* (eds. Whelpton and Kiser), **III**, *Milbank Memorial Fund* (New York, 1953).
12 R. Gopalswami in *Research in Family Planning* (ed. Kiser) (Princeton, 1962).

Chapter 5

1 E. L. Bernstein, *Hum. Fert.* **5** (1940).
2 *Boswell's London Journal, 1762–1763* (London: Yale Edition, 1950).
3 N. Himes, *Medical History of Contraception* (New York, 1936).
4 *The Machine* (London, 1744).
5 E. J. Dingwall, *Br. Med. J.* **1** (1953).
6 C. I. B. Voge, *The Chemistry and Physics of Contraception* (London, 1933).
7 British Standards Institution *Specification for Rubber Condoms*, BS 3704, 1964 (London, 1964).
8 *Fifth Public Opinion Survey on Birth Control in Japan* (Tokyo, 1961).
9 M. Peberdy in *Biological Aspects of Social Problems* (eds. Meade and Parkes) (Edinburgh, 1965).
10 Economist Intelligence Unit, *Retail Business* (1965).
11 H. Rattner, *J. Am. Med. Ass.* (1935).
12 A. Stone, *International Birth Control Conference Report* (Zurich, 1930).
13 W. H. Masters & V. E. Johnson, *Human Sexual Response* (London, 1966).
14 C. Tietze, *Advances in Sex Research* (New York, 1963).
15 IPPF *Med. Bull.* **2**, 1 February 1968.

Chapter 6

1 J. Casanova, *The Memoirs of Jacques Casanova de Seingalt* (London: Navarre Edition, 1922).
2 F. A. Wilde, *Das Weibliche Gebar-Unvermoaen* (Berlin, 1838).

3 *Lancet*, vol. II (1867).
4 D. M. Mensinga, *Fakultative Sterilat* (Leipzig, 1882).
5 F. Lafitte, *Family Planning in the Sixties* (Birmingham, 1963).
6 R. Freedman, P. K. Whelpton & A. A. Campbell, *Family Planning, Sterility and Population Growth* (New York, 1959).
7 R. M. Pierce & G. Rowntree, *Popul. Stud.* **15** (1961).
8 C. F. Westoff & N. B. Ryder, *Studies in Family Planning*, **17** (1967).
9 C. F. Westoff, R. G. Potter & P. C. Sagi, *The Third Child* (Princeton, 1963).
10 J. & E. Newson, *Patterns of Infant Care in an Urban Community* (London, 1963).
11 P. E. Treffers, *Popul. Stud.* **20** (1967).

Chapter 7

1 J. Peel, *Popul. Stud.* **16** (1962).
2 M. Woodside & E. Slater, *Patterns of Working Class Marriages* (London, 1947).
3 M. Stopes, *Contraception* (London, 1947).
4 'Contraceptives', *Which?* Supplement (London, 1967).
5 G. Rowntree & R. M. Pierce, *Popul. Stud.* **15** (1961).
6 'Contraceptives', *Which?* Supplement (London, 1966).
7 *The Population Council 1952–1964*, A Report (1965).
8 J. T. Dingle & C. Tietze, *Am. J. Obstet. Gynec.* **85** (1963).
9 E. Mears & N. W. Please, *J. Reprod. Fert.* **3** (1962).
10 H. M. Husein, *Proceedings of the U.N. World Population Conference* (New York, 1967).
11 E. Mears, *J. Reprod. Fert.* **4** (1962).

Chapter 8

1 N. E. Himes, *Medical History of Contraception* (Baltimore, 1936).
2 J. T. Noonan, *Contraception* (Cambridge, Mass., 1965).
3 H. Knaus, *Zentbl. Gynäk.* **53** (1929).
4 K. Ogino, *Zentbl. Gynäk.* **56** (1931).
5 E. Allen, J. P. Pratt, Q. V. Newell & L. J. Bland, *Contrib. Embryol.* (Washington, 1930).
6 R. Freedman, P. K. Whelpton & A. A. Campbell, *Family Planning, Sterility and Population Growth* (New York, 1959).
7 G. Rowntree & R. Pierce, *Popul. Stud.* **15** (1961).
8 *Studies in Family Planning*, no. 17 (1967).
9 J. Peel, *The Hull Marriage Survey: Some Preliminary Findings*, in press.
10 J. Marshall, *Planning for a Family* (London, 1965).
11 L. Iffy, *J. Obstet. Gynaec. Br. Commonw.* **68** (1961).
12 R. G. Cross, *Br. Med. J.* **3**, 27 July 1968.
13 Quoted in J. Rock, *The Time Has Come* (London, 1963).
14 A. J. de Bethune, *Science*, **142** (1963).

Chapter 9

1 D. W. MacCorquodale, S. A. Thayer & E. A. Doisy, *J. Biol. Chem.* **115** (1936).
2 S. H. Sturgis & F. Albright, *Endocrinology*, **26** (1940).
3 J. Rock, G. Pincus & C. R. Carcia, *Science*, **124** (1956).
4 J. W. Goldzieher, J. Martin-Manautau & N. B. Livingston, *West. J. Surg. Obstet. Gynec.* **71** (1963).
5 S. Zuckerman (ed.), *The Ovary* (New York, 1962).
6 A. S. Parkes (ed.), *Marshall's Physiology of Reproduction* (London, 1966).
7 J. A. Loraine & T. E. Bell, *Fertility and Contraception in the Human Female* (Edinburgh, 1968).
8 F. B. Colton & P. D. Klimstra in *Encyclopedia of Chemical Technology* (New York, 1965).
9 G. T. Ross, W. D. Odell & P. L. Rayford, *Lancet*, **2** (1966).
10 J. Zanartu, *Int. J. Fert.* **9** (1964).
11 F. J. Saunders, *Endocrinology*, **77** (1965).
12 E. Mears (ed.), *Handbook of Oral Contraception* (London, 1965).
13 V. A. Drill, *Oral Contraceptives* (New York, 1966).
14 G. Pincus, *The Control of Fertility* (New York, 1965).
15 G. Pincus, C. R. Garcia & J. Rock, *Science*, **130** (1959).
16 K. Dalton, *The Premenstrual Syndrome* (London, 1964).
17 A. Wiseman, *Br. med. J.* **2** (1963).
18 J. A. Zadeh, C. D. Karabus & J. Fielding, *Br. med. J.* **4** (1967).
19 J. S. Strauss & P. E. Pouchi in *Ovulation* (ed. Greenblatt) (Philadelphia, 1966).
20 J. E. Murphy, *Clin. Trials J.* **5** (1968).
21 E. C. G. Grant, *Br. med. J.* **2** (1968).
22 J. Lindhe & A. L. Bjorn, *J. Peridont. Res.* **2** (1967).
23 W. H. Jordan, *Lancet*, **2** (1961).
24 Food and Drug Administration Report on Enovid. (See also *J. Am. med. Ass.* **185**, 1963.)
25 Subcommittee of the Medical Research Council, *Br. med. J.* **2** (1967).
26 W. H. W. Inman & M. P. Vessey, *Br. med. J.* **2** (1968).
27 M. P. Vessey & R. Doll, *Br. med. J.* **2** (1968).
28 R. L. Holmes & A. M. Mandl, *Lancet*, **1** (1962).
29 A. B. Kar, H. Chandra, V. P. Kamboj & S. R. Chowdhury, *Indian J. exp. Biol.* **3** (1965).
30 R. P. Shearman, *Lancet*, **2** (1966).
31 E. Johannisson, K. G. Tillinger & E. Diczfalusy, *Fert. Steril.* **16** (1963).
32 C. J. Meyer, D. S. Layne, J. F. Tait & G. Pincus, *J. clin. Invest.* **40** (1961).
33 G. I. M. Swyer & V. Little, *Br. med. J.* **1** (1965).
34 V. Larsen-Cohn, *Br. med. J.* **1** (1965).
35 J. S. Allan & E. T. Tyler, *Fert. Steril.* **18** (1967).
36 V. Wynn & J. W. H. Doar, *Lancet*, **2** (1966).

37 V. Wynn, J. W. H. Doar & G. L. Mills, *Lancet*, **2** (1966).
38 A. D. Satterthwaite & C. J. Gamble, *J. Am. Med. Wom. Ass.* **17** (1962).
39 B. D. Jacobsen, *Am. J. Obstet. Gynec.* **84** (1962).
40 B. D. Jacobsen, *Acta endocr. Copenh.* **45** (1964).
41 D. H. Carr, *Lancet*, **2** (1967).
42 *Wld. Hlth. Org. techn. Rep. Ser.* **386** (WHO, Geneva, 1968).
43 R. A. Wilson, *J. Am. med. Ass.* **182** (1962).
44 J. A. Larson, *Obstet. Gynecol.* **3** (1954).
45 E. Rice-Wray, J. W. Goldzieher & A. Aranda-Rosell, *Fert. Steril.* **14** (1963).
46 I.P.P.F. *Med. Bull.* **2**, (1969).
47 V. Gellman, *Manitoba med. Rev.* **44** (1964).
48 A. Sharman, *Clin. Trials J.* **5** (1968).
49 R. B. Greenblatt, *Med. Sci.* **37** (1967).
50 T. Kaern, *Br. med. J.* **3** (1967).
51 G. Pincus & G. R. Garcia, in *Recent Advances in Ovarian and Synthetic Steroids* (ed. Shearman) (Sydney, 1965).

Chapter 10

1 J. Casanova, *The Memoirs of Jacques Casanova de Seingalt* (London: Navarre Edition, 1922).
2 A. Guttmacher, *Family Planning*, **13** (1965).
3 E. Grafenberg, *Third Congress of World League for Sexual Reform* (London, 1929).
4 A. Stone & N. E. Himes, *Practical Birth Control Methods* (London, 1960).
5 H. Kondo, *Japan Parenthood Quarterly* (January–March 1953).
6 A. Ishihama, *Yokohama Medical Bulletin*, 1959.
7 W. A. Bonney, S. R. Glasser, T. H. Clewe, R. W. Noyes & C. L. Cooper, *Am. J. Obstet. Gynec.* **96** (1966).
8 L. Mastroianni & C. H. Rosseau, *J. Obstet. Gynaec.* **93** (1965).
9 C. Tietze, *Proceedings of the Fifth World Congress on Fertility and Sterility*, *Excerpta Medica*, International Conference Series, **133** (New York, 1967).
10. W. A. Kelly & J. H. Marston, *Nature*, **214** (1967).
11 A. Psychoyos & V. Bitten, *C.R. Séanc. Soc. Biol.* **160** (1965).
12 A. B. Kar, V. P. Kamboj, A. Goswami & S. R. Chowdhury, *J. Reprod. Fert.* **9** (1965).
13 H. M. Carlton & H. J. Phelps, *J. Obstet. Gynaec. Br. Emp.* **40** (1933).
14 M. Potts & R. M. Pearson, *J. Obstet. Gynaec. Br. Commonw.* **74** (1967).
15 F. Szontagh, L. Zelenka & Z. Szereday, *Preventive Medicine and Family Planning*, IPPF (London, 1966).
16 *Leviticus*, **15**, 1–33.
17 G. A. Liss & G. T. Andros, *Am. J. Obstet. Gynec.* **94** (1966).
18 L. Andolsek, *Proceedings of the Eighth International Conference of the International Planned Parenthood Federation*, IPPF (London, 1967).

19 *Wld. Hlth. Org. techn. Rep. Ser.* **332** (Geneva, 1966).
20 L. Hallberg, A. M. Högdahl, L. Nilsson & G. Rybo, *Acta obstet. gynec. scand.* **45** (1966).
21 J. A. Zadeh, C. D. Karabus & J. Fielding, *Br. med. J.* **4** (1967).
22 J. Lippes, *Am. J. Obstet. Gynec.* **93** (1965).
23 E. Rosen, *Am. J. Obstet. Gynec.* **93** (1965).
24 R. Ansbacher, W. A. Boyson & J. A. Morris, *Am. J. Obstet. Gynec.* **99** (1967).
25 D. R. Mishell, J. H. Bell, R. G. Good & D. L. Moyer, *Am. J. Obstet. Gynec.* **96** (1966).
26 C. Tietze, *Am. J. Obstet. Gynec.* **96** (1966).
27 J. Thambu, *Br. med. J.* **2** (1965).

Chapter 11

1 N. E. Himes, *Medical History of Contraception* (London, 1936 and 1963).
2 M. Stopes, *Contraception* (London, 1949).
3 A. C. Kinsey, W. B. Pomeroy, C. E. Martin & P. H. Gebhard, *Sexual Behaviour in the Human Female* (Philadelphia and London, 1953).
4 E. Gautier & L. Henry, *La Population de Crulai, Paroisse Normande* (Paris, 1958).
5 C. Tietze, *Proceedings of the International Population Conference*, vol. 2 (New York, 1961).
6 D. Robinson & J. Rock, *Obstet. Gynec.* **29** (1967).

Chapter 12

1 C. P. Blacker, *Eugen. Rev.* **53** (1961).
2 A. A. Campbell, *Am. J. Obstet. Gynec.* **89** (1964).
3 D. Baird, *Contraception Control*, Excerpta Medica Foundation (1966).
4 T. Lu & D. Chun, *J. Obstet. Gynaec. Br. Commonw.* **74** (1967).
5 A. S. Ferber, C. Tietze & S. Lewit, *Psychosom. Med.* **29** (1967).
6 M. Madlener, *Zentralbt. f. Gynäk.* **20** (1919).
7 P. C. Steptoe, *Br. med. J.* **1** (1966).
8 S. Yasui, *Jap. Med. J.* **1475** (1952).
9 H. Boysen, L. A. McRae & N. M. Albuguerque, *Am. J. Obstet. Gynec.* **58** (1949).
10 R. E. Bieren & J. M. Hundley, *Am. J. Obstet. Gynec.* **54** (1947).
11 D. B. Rees, *Am. J. Obstet. Gynec.* **82** (1961).
12 A. M. Phadke, *J. Reprod. Fert.* **7** (1964).
13 A. M. Phadke & K. Padukone, *J. Reprod. Fert.* **7** (1964).
14 H. J. Roberts, *J. Am. Geriat. Soc.* **16** (1968).
15 W. N. Thornton & T. J. Williams, *Am. J. Obstet. Gynec.* **42** (1941).
16 C. B. Lull, *Pennsylvania M.J.* **43** (1940).
17 S. S. Schmidt, *Fert. Steril.* **17** (1966).
18 T. W. Adams, *Am. J. Obstet. Gynec.* **89** (1954).
19 F. Jensen & J. Lester, *Acta obst. et gynec. scand.* **36** (1957).

20 N. Chaset, *J. Urol.* **87** (1962).
21 B. Thompson & D. Baird, *Lancet*, **1** (1968).
22 P. Barglow & M. Eisner, *Am. J. Obstet. Gynec.* **95** (1966).
23 D. A. Rogers, F. I. Ziegler & M. Levy, *Psychosom. Med.* **29** (1967).
24 M. H. Johnson, *Amer. J. Psychiat.* **121** (1964).
25 A. C. Barnes & F. P. Zuspan, *Am. J. Obstet. Gynec.* **75** (1958).
26 F. J. Ziegler, D. A. Rogers & S. A. Kriegsman, *Psychosom. Med.* **28** (1966).
27 W. J. Dieckmann & E. B. Hauser, *Am. J. Obstet. Gynec.* **55** (1948).
28 G. M. & A. G. Phadke, *J. Urol.* **97** (1967).
29 W. C. W. Nixon, *Proc. R. Soc. Med.* **50** (1957).

Chapter 13

1 R. G. Potter, J. B. Wyon, M. New & J. E. Gordon, *Hum. Biol.* **37** (1965).
2 S. Shapiro, E. W. Jones & P. M. Denson, *Milbank Meml. Fund Q.* **40** (1962).
3 A. T. Hertig, J. Rock, E. C. Adams & M. F. Menkin, *Pediatrics*, **28** (1959).
4 M. Kerr, M. N. Rashad, S. Christie & A. Ross, *Am. J. Obstet. Gynec.* **94** (1966).
5 P. M. Gebhard, W. B. Pomeroy, C. E. Martin & C. V. Christenson, *Pregnancy, Birth and Abortion* (New York, 1958).
6 M. Potts, *Eugen. Rev.* **59** (1968).
7 T. N. Parish, *J. Obstet. Gynaec. Br. Commonw.* **42** (1935).
8 P. P. Bricknell, H. G. Middleton, A. Hollingsworth & E. M. C. Evans, *Br. med. J.* **2**, 400 (1967).
9 P. Rhodes in *Abortion in Britain* (London, 1966).
10 M. Forssman & I. Thume, *Acta Psychiat. neurol. scand.* **42** (1966).
11 T. F. Pugh, B. K. Jerath, W. M. Schmidt & R. B. Reed, *New Engl. J. Med.* **268**, 1.
12 E. W. Anderson, *J. Ment. Sci.* **79** (1933).
13 C. M. McLane in *Abortion in the United States* (ed. M. S. Calderone) (New York, 1958).
14 E. Tylden, *Med. Wld.* **104** (1966).
15 G. af Geijerstam in *Abortion in the United States* (ed. M. S. Calderone) (New York, 1958).
16 M. E. Martin, *Br. med. J.* **2** (1958).
17 N. Butler & D. G. Bonham, *Perinatal Mortality* (Edinburgh, 1963).
18 T. McKeown, R. G. Record, in *Ciba Foundation Symposium on Congenital Malformations* (ed. G. E. W. Wolstenholm) (London, 1960).
19 E. M. Hare, K. M. Lawrence, H. Paynes & K. Rawnsley, *Br. med. J.* **2** (1966).
20 *Human Genetics*, Ministry of Health (London, 1967).
21 M. S. Adams & J. V. Neal, *Pediatrics* (Springfield), **40** (1967).
22 D. F. Roberts, *Br. med. J.* **2** (1967).

23 *Rubella and other Virus Infections in Pregnancy*, Ministry of Health Report on Public Health and Medical Subjects, **101** (London, 1960).
24 M. D. Sheridan, *Br. med. J.* **2** (1964).
25 I. Leck, *Br. J. prev. soc. Med.* **17** (1963).
26 J. O. Shone, S. M. Armas, J. A. Manning & J. D. Keith, *Pediatrics*, **37** (1966).
27 A. B. Hill, R. Doll, T. McL. Galloway & J. P. W. Hughes, *Br. J. prev. soc. Med.* **12** (1958).
28 E. B. Shaw & H. L. Steinbeck, *Am. J. Dis. Child.* **115** (1968).
29 G. L. Muller & S. Graham, *New Engl. J. Med.* **252** (1955).
30 Report by the BMA Committee on Therapeutic Abortion, *Br. med. J.* **1** (1968).
31 B. MacMahon, *J. natn. Cancer Inst.* **28** (1962).
32 T. N. A. Jeffcoate, *Br. med. J.* **1** (1960).
33 C. S. Burwell & J. Metcalfe, *Heart Disease and Pregnancy* (London, 1958).
34 A. R. Gilchrist, *Br. med. J.* **1** (1963).
35 L. Williams, *Br. med. J.* **2** (1957).
36 C. W. Manning, F. J. Prime & P. A. Zorab, *Lancet*, **2** (1967).
37 J. Peel, *Br. med. J.* **2** (1955).
38 Y. T. & H. C. Wu, *Chin. J. Obstet. Gynec.* **6** (1958).
39 D. Kerslake & D. Casey, *Obstet. Gynec.* **30** (1967).
40 Y. T. Wu & L. M. Shang, *Chin. J. Obstet. Gynec.* **11** (1965).
41 E. Holland, *Proc. R. Soc. Med.* **26** (1932).
42 E. Aburel, Communicare la Sociecatea Stiintelor Medicale, Iasi. (1934).
43 J. M. Cameron & A. D. Dayan, *Br. med. J.* **1** (1966).
44 T. Wagatsuma, *Am. J. Obstet. Gynec.* **93** (1965).
45 R. W. Weilerstein, *J. Am. Med. Ass.* **125** (1944).
46 J. B. Thiersch, *Am. J. Obstet. Gynec.* **63** (1952).
47 K. H. Mehlan in *Proc. VII Conf. IPPF*, Excerpta Medica Foundation (Int. Conf. Series, **72**) (Amsterdam, 1964).
48 G. Topp, *Zentbl. Gynäk.* **81** (1959).
49 A. Černoch, *Čslká. Gynek.* **25** (1960).
50 J. Lindahl, *Somatic Complications following Legal Abortion* (Stockholm, 1959).
51 H. G. Berthelsen, E. Ostergaard, *Dan. Med. Bull.* **6** (1959).
52 E. Vladov, I. Ivanov, A. Angelov & I. Rakilovska, *Gynaecologia*, **159** (1965).
53 G. L. Timanus in *Abortion in the United States* (ed. Calderone) (New York, 1958).
54 G. Winter, *Die Künstliche Schwangerschaftsunterbreching*, Enke-Verlag (Stuttgart, 1949).
55 J. Gellen, Z. Zovacs, F. E. Szontagh & D. Boda, *Br. med. J.* **2** (1965).
56 N. M. Simon & A. G. Senturia, *Archs. Gen. Psychiat.* **15** (1966).
57 R. B. White, *Tex. Rep. Biol. Med.* **24** (1966).
58 M. Ekblad, *Acta Psychiat. neurol. scand.* Suppl. **99** (1955).
59 O. Kolarova, J. Stanicek & G. Jicinska, *Geburtshierflich-Gynaekolosische Gesellschaft*, **60** (1966).

Chapter 14

1 *Television Act*, 1954, Sect. 4(5), and Independent Television Authority, *Principles of Television Advertising* (London, 1960).
2 M. A. Pyke, *Eugen. Rev.* **55** (1963).
3 *National Health Service: the administrative structure of medical and related services in England and Wales* (HMSO, London, 1968).
4 L. Corsa, *Studies in Family Planning*, **27** (1968).
5 Legal correspondent, *Br. med. J.* (19 November 1960).
6 G. Williams, *The Sanctity of Life and the Criminal Law* (London, 1958).
7 M. S. Calderone (ed.), *Abortion in the United States* (New York, 1958).
8 H. Rosen, *Abortion in America* (New York, 1967).
9 H. Packer & R. Gampell, *Stanford Law Review*, **11** (1959).
10 J. B. Gardner in *British Obstetric and Gynaecological Practice* (eds. Holland and Bourne) (London, 1955).
11 P. M. Addison, *Med.-lag. J.* **35** (1967).
12 M. Sanger, *My Fight for Birth Control* (London, 1932).
13 L. N. Jackson, *Family Planning*, **15** (1966).
14 K. Hindle & M. Simms, *Pol. Q.* **39** (1968).

Chapter 15

1 D. A. Boyes, H. K. Fidler & D. R. Lock, *Br. med. J.* **1** (1962).
2 M. Schofield, *The Sexual Behaviour of Young People* (London, 1965).
3 D. Wallace, *Am. J. Obstet. Gynec.* **92** (1965).
4 A. F. Clift, *Proc. Roy. Soc. Med.* **39** (1945).
5 T. Sato & R. B. Greenblatt, *Am. J. Obstet. Gynec.* **89** (1965).
6 C. L. Buxton & A. L. Southam, *Human Infertility* (London, 1958).
7 M. M. White & V. B. Green-Armytage, *The Management of Impaired Fertility* (London, 1962).
8 R. W. Noyes & E. M. Chapnick, *Fertil. Steril.* **15** (1964).
9 J. P. Jacobs, *J. Iowa Med. Soc.* **3** (1965).

Chapter 16

1 B. Benjamin, *Health and Vital Statistics* (London, 1968).
2 Ministry of Health, *Report on Confidential Enquiry into Maternal Death in England and Wales 1958–1960* (HMSO, London, 1963).
3 WHO *Report* (1963).
4 J. W. B. Douglas & C. Mogford, *Br. med. J.* **1** (1953).
5 J. W. B. Douglas, *Br. med. J.* **1** (1956).
6 C. M. Drillien & F. Richmond, *Archs. Dis. Childh.* **31** (1956).
7 N. R. Butler & D. G. Bonham, *Perinatal Mortality* (Edinburgh, 1963).
8 J. A. Heady, C. Daley & J. N. Morris, *Lancet*, **1** (1955).
9 J. K. Russell, D. V. I. Fairweather, D. G. M. Millar, A. M. Brown, R. C. M. Pearson, G. A. Neligan, & G. S. Anderson, *Lancet*, **1** (1963).
10 *Children in Care in England and Wales* (HMSO, London, 1967).

11 K. Soddy in *Sex and Human Relations* (IPPF, London, 1965).

12 A. C. Fraser & P. S. Watson, *Practitioner*, **201** (1968).

13 C. F. Westoff, R. G. Potter & P. C. Sagi, *The Third Child* (Princeton, 1963).

14 R. Freedman, P. K. Whelpton & A. A. Campbell, *Family Planning, Sterility and Population Growth* (New York, 1959).

15 *Circumstances of Families* (HMSO, London, 1967).

16 E. H. Hare & G. K. Shaw, *Br. J. Psychiat.* **3** (1965).

17 M. Stopes, *Roman Catholic Methods of Birth Control* (London, 1923).

18 R. E. Dowse & J. Peel, *Pol. Stud.* **13** (1965).

19 *Lancet*, **1** (1959).

20 A. Cartwright, *Med. Offcr.* **120** (19 July 1968).

21 V. A. Drill, *Oral Contraceptives* (New York, 1966).

22 G. Pincus, *The Control of Fertility* (New York, 1965).

23 C. R. Austin & J. S. Perry (eds.), *Agents Affecting Fertility* (London, 1965).

24 M. Jackson, *Antifertility Compounds in the Male and Female* (Springfield, 1966).

25 Current references to this rapidly expanding field can be found in the *Bibliography of Reproduction*, Reproduction Research Information Services Ltd, Cambridge.

26 E. T. Tyler in *Proceedings of the Eighth International Conference of the International Planned Parenthood Federation* (London, 1967).

27 H. Bruce, *J. Reprod. Fert.* **4** (1962).

28 J. Martin-Manautau, J. Giner Velázquez, R. Aznar-Ramos, M. Lozano-Balderas & W. H. Rudel in *Proceedings of the Eighth International Conference of the International Planned Parenthood Federation*, IPPF (London, 1967).

29 J. Zañartu, M. Pupkin, D. Rosenberg, R. Gueffero, R. Rodriguez-Bravo, M. Garcia-Huidobro & A. Puga, *Br. med. J.* **2** (1968).

30 J. McLean Morris & G. Van Wagenen in *Proceedings of the Eighth International Conference of the International Planned Parenthood Federation*, IPPF (London, 1967).

31 R. M. Moore & L. E. A. Rowson, *J. Reprod. Fert.* **12** (1966).

32 L. Engstrom, *IPPF Med. Bull.* **2** (1968).

33 C. G. Heller, D. J. Moore & C. A. Paulsen, *Toxic. apl. Pharmac.* **3** (1961).

34 H. Jackson, B. W. Fox & A. W. Craig, *J. Reprod. Fert.* **2** (1961).

35 K. Landsteiner, *Zentbl. Bakt. Parasitkde*, **25** (1899).

36 P. R. Cox, *Demography*, 4th edition (London, 1969).

37 *U.N. Working Group on Social Demography—Report* (Geneva, 1967).

38 *IPPF News*, **164** (1967).

39 *New Scient.* **39** (1968).

References to figures and tables

The sources of data used in most of the figures and tables are indicated in the text; others are based on vital statistics obtained from the United Nations *Demographic Yearbooks* or from other official publications such as the Registrar General's *Statistical Reviews for England and Wales*. The origin of data used in the remaining figures and tables is shown below.

Fig. 2   Adapted from N. E. Himes & V. C. Himes, *Hosp. Soc. Serv.* **19**, (1929) and F. Lafitte, *Family Planning in the Sixties* (Birmingham, 1963).

Fig. 6   C. F. Westoff & N. B. Ryder, *Studies in Family Planning* **17** (1967).

Fig. 22   J. A. Loraine, E. T. Bell, R. A. Harkness, E. Mears & M. C. N. Jackson, *Lancet* **2** (1963).

Figs. 23 and 24   G. Pincus, *The Control of Fertility* (New York, 1965).

Fig. 27   Personal communication from R. Barnard, The Pathfinder Fund, 1968.

Fig. 29   C. Tietze, A. F. Guttmacher & S. Rubin, *J. Am. med. Ass.* **142** (1950).

Fig. 30   P. H. Gebhard, W. B. Pomeroy, C. F. Martin & C. V. Christensen, *Pregnancy, Birth and Abortion* (New York, 1958); C. Tietze & C. F. Martin, *Popul. St.* **11** (1951); E. K. Brunner, *Human Biol.* **13** (1941).

Fig. 31   P. H. Gebhard, W. B. Pomeroy, C. F. Martin & C. V. Christensen, *Pregnancy, Birth and Abortion* (New York, 1958).

Fig. 32   M. Potts, *Eugen. Rev.* **59** (1968).

Figs. 33 and 34   Ministry of Health, *Rubella and Other Virus Infections in Pregnancy*, Public Health and Medical Subjects, **101** (1960).

Fig. 36   M. Potts, *Eugen. Rev.* **59** (1968).

Fig. 37   C. Muller & M. Mall-Haefele, *Medic. Gynaec. and Sociol.* **3** (1968).

Fig. 38   Constructed from a large number of demographic and sociological investigations.

Fig. 39   SPBCC and FPA Annual Reports.

Table 5   J. d'A. Jeffery & A. I. Klopper, *J. Reprod. Fertil.*, Suppl. **4** (1968).

Table 6   A. Wiseman, *Recent Advances in Ovarian and Synthetic Steroids* (ed. Shearman) (Sidney, 1965).

Table 7   W. H. W. Inman & M. P. Vessey, *Br. Med. J.* **2** (1968).

Table 9   C. Tietze, *Am. J. Obstet. Gynec.* **96** (1966) and *Cooperative Statistical Program for Evaluation of Intrauterine Devices* (New York, 1966); K. Frith, *Br. Med. J.* **2** (1967); M. H. Knock, *Am. J. Obstet. Gynec.* **99** (1967); A. Goldenstein, *Proceedings of the Fifth World Congress on Fertility and Sterility, Excerpta Medica* **133** (1967); F. Zontagh, Personal communication, 1968; J. Sracek, J. Autos, O. Blaskove *et al. Cslka Gynek* **32** (1967).

Tables 10 and 11   C. Tietze, *Am. J. Obstet. Gynec.* **96** (1966).

Table 12   A. S. Ferber, C. Tietze & S. Lewit, *Psychosom. Med.* **29** (1967).

Table 13   A. E. Garb, *Obstet. Gynec. Survey* **12** (1957).

Table 14   W. J. Dieckmann & E. B. Hauser, *Am. J. Obstet. Gynec.* **55** (1948).

Tables 15 and 16   H. Forsman & I. Thurne, *Acta Psychiat. neurol. Scand.* **42** (1966).

Table 19   A. R. Gilchrist, *Br. med. J.* **1** (1963).

Table 20   Y. Moriyasna, *Harmful Effects of Induced Abortion* (Tokyo, 1966); F. Novak, *Preventive Medicine and Family Planning, Excerpta Medica* (1966); A. Cernoch, *Gynecologia,* **160** (1965); K. H. Mehlan, *Family Planning and Population Programs* (ed. Berelson) (Chicago, 1966).

Table 21   A. Klinger, *Family Planning and Population Programs* (ed. Berelson) (Chicago, 1966).

Table 23   B. Benjamin, *Health and Vital Statistics* (London, 1968).

Table 24   A. Cartwright, *Med. Offr.* **120** (1968).

Index

abortifacients, 200, 258
abortion, 159, 169 ff, 243
  criminal, 173, 174, 224, 243
  death rate: criminal, 174, 243, 253; therapeutic, 203, 253
  definition, 169
  eugenic indications, 182 ff; genetic, 183, 184; radiation, 188, 189; rhesus incompatibility, 189; teratogenic drugs, 187, 188; viral agents and diseases, 186
  evaluation, 208, 209
  incidence: induced, 23, 172, 224; spontaneous, 145, 169, 170
  legislation, 217 ff, 222, 223, 224
  medical indications: abdominal emergencies, 194; chorea gravidarium, 193; diabetes, 192; heart diseases, 190, 191; incapacitating diseases, 194; kidney diseases, 192; malignancy, 193; obstetric and gynaecological conditions, 193, 194; otosclerosis, 193; phaeochromocytoma, 193; pulmonary hypertension, 191; syphilis, 194; tuberculosis, 191
  methods: abortifacient drugs, 200, 258, 259; abortifacient paste, 200; dilatation and curettage, 195, 196, 201 ff; hysterotomy, 197, 198; intra-amniotic injections, 199, 200; uterine aspiration, 196, 197; with sterilization, 159
  psychiatric indications: endogenous depression, 181; immaturity, 182; manic depression, 182; mental defect, 182; previous puerperal psychosis, 181; psychopathy, 182; reactive depression, 180, 181; schizophrenia, 181, 182; suicide and threat of suicide, 181
  role in family planning, 23, 175, 224, 251
  side effects: medical and surgical, 201–205; psychological, 205, 206; social, 206, 208
  social indications: the child, 177, 178; the mother, 176, 177; the unmarried, 178; 'total environment', 175
Abortion Law Reform Association, 225

advice to the unmarried, 233
aerosols, *see* chemical contraceptives
age at marriage, 31, 32, 233
American College of Obstetricians, 16, 17
American Medical Association, 15
American Public Health Association, 17
American Society for the Study of sterility, 237, 240
aminopterin, 188, 200
Anovlar, 92, 101, 121
Anovlar-21, 92, 121
Antigon, 134
asthma, 125

battered babies, 246
being careful, *see* coitus interruptus
Birnberg bow, 133, 144, 145
birth control clinics, 7, 11, 12, 14, 26, 28, 29, 43, 44, 59, 61, 62, 75
Birth Control Investigation Committee, 11, 12, 13, 16, 36, 37
birth rates
  Chile, 30
  Egypt, 30
  England and Wales, 19
  Mauritius, 30
  U.S.A., 245
Bradlaugh–Besant trial, 4, 5, 21, 22
breakthrough bleeding, 90, 118, 121
breast discomfort, 106
breast enlargement, 106, 120
breastfeeding, 122, 123, 151, 152
British Medical Association, 6, 14, 15, 128, 220
British Standards Institution, 39, 40, 56

Caesarean Section, 158, 159, 163, 167, 198, 202
cancer, 115, 125, 132, 193
candida albicans, 228
castration, 153, 160
census of England and Wales, 18, 21
cervical cytology, 38, 116, 119, 157, 230, 231
cervicitis, 227

INDEX

intrauterine device (*cont.*)
  distortion within uterus, 133
  efficacy, 130
  evaluation, 146, 147, 148
  expulsion, 133, 138, 143
  extent of use, 148
  failure rates, 137
  follow-up, 141
  Grafenberg ring, 129
  history, 128
  in monkey experiments, 131
  in primitive society, 128
  in rodent experiments, 131, 132
  insertion, 135, 136, 137, 138, 139, 140
  introducers, 134, 140
  long term effects, 132, 251, 254
  mode of action, 129, 130, 131
  patents, 215
  removal, 146
  risk of perforation, 133, 144
  side effects, 129: bleeding, 142; death, 129, 141, 142, 251; endometritis, 129; expulsion, 143; infection, 144; pain, 143; pelvic inflammation, 129; perforation, 144; peritonitis, 129; pregnancy, 145; septicaemia, 129
  storage and sterilization, 135, 138
  subsequent pregnancies, 146
  testing, 40
  types available, 133, 134
  wishbones and collarstuds, 128, 129

Japan
  population policies, 33, 56, 129, 210, 219, 224
Jews, and periodic abstinence, 87, 137

lactation, 87, 122, 123, 146, 151, 152
law
  effectiveness, 222, 223, 224
  function, 210
  on abortion, 175, 217 ff; Eastern Europe, 175, 219; England, 175, 217; Germany, 219; Japan, 219; Scandinavia, 175, 219; United States, 218; U.S.S.R., 219
  on contraception, 211 ff; Denmark, 214; Eastern Europe, 214; England, 211, 212; France, 214; Germany, 215; United States, 212, 213, 214; U.S.S.R., 215
  on sterilization, 215 ff; Denmark, 217; England, 215, 216; India, 217; Puerto Rico, 217; Sweden, 217; United States, 216
  patent, 215

Lippes loop, 133, 140, 144
luteinizing hormone (LH), 91, 98, 130, 239
Lyndiol, 92, 95, 121
Lyndiol-2·5, 92, 95, 121
Lynestrenol, 95

Madlener technique, 158, 165
Malthusian League, 4, 6, 10, 22
Margaret Sanger Research Bureau, 38
Margulies spiral, 133, 144
maternal morbidity, 242 ff
maternal mortality, 7, 174, 242, 243
M-device, 133
Medical Defence Union, 216
medical education, 15
Medical Research Council, 109
medroxyprogesterone acetate, 94
megestrol acetate, 94
menopause, 87, 124, 142
menstruation, 103, 104, 142
Mestranol, 92, 103
Ministry of Health, 13, 211, 212, 230, 248
Minovlar, 121
mittelschmerz, 105, 238
mortality and morbidity, contraceptive, 5, 10, 51, 108, 141, 161, 174, 203, 251 ff
Moslems, 137
multiple sclerosis, 125, 194
mythology of contraception, 35, 52, 73

National Birth Rate Commission, 6, 7, 11, 36
National Committee on Maternal Health, 36
nineteenth-century birth control movement, 2, 3
Noracyclin, 121
norethisterone (=norethindrone), 89, 95, 119
norethisterone acetate (=norethindrone acetate), 95
Norethynodrel, 90, 96
Norgestrel, 95
Norlestrin, 95, 97, 121
Norlestrin-21, 95, 121
Norinyl-1, 95, 97, 121, 122
Nuvacon, 97, 121

obesity, 126
oestradiol, 91
Oneida Community, 150
Oracon, 96
oral contraceptives, 89 ff, 252 ff
  accidental swallowing by children, 119
  acne, 104
  alopecia, 106

INDEX